the **ayurvedic** year

the **ayurvedic** year

christina**brown**

**STOREY
BOOKS**

The mission of Storey Publishing is to serve our customers by publishing practical information that encourages personal independence in harmony with the environment.

United States edition published in 2002 by Storey Books, 210 MASS MoCA Way, North Adams, MA 01247

United Kingdom edition published in 2002 by MQ Publications Ltd, 12 The Ivories, 6-8 Northampton Street, London N1 2HY

Editor: Kate John, MQ Publications Ltd; Jennifer Travis Donnelly, Storey Publishing
Editorial Director: Ljiljana Baird, MQ Publications Ltd; Deborah Balmuth, Storey Publishing
Art Direction: John Casey, MQ Publications Ltd; Meredith Maker, Storey Publishing
Illustrator: Penny Brown

The information in this book is true and complete to the best of our knowledge. All recommendations are made without guarantee on the part of the author or Storey Books. The author and publisher disclaim any liability in connection with the use of this information. For additional information please contact Storey Books, 210 MASS MoCA Way, North Adams, MA 01247.

Printed in China

Library of Congress Cataloging-in-Publication Data

Brown, Christina
The ayurvedic year: a seasonal guide to nutrition, yoga, and healing / by Christina Brown.
p. cm.
ISBN 1-58017-444-2 (alk. paper)
1. Medicine, Ayurvedic. I. Title.

R605 B76 2002
615.53—dc21

2001055132

Publisher's note: This publication is intended to provide educational information for the reader on the covered subject. It is not intended to take the place of personalized medical counseling, diagnosis and treatment from a trained health professional.

contents

what is ayurveda?

Ayurveda is a complete holistic medical system that has been practiced in India for thousands of years. In the ancient language of Sanskrit, *ayus* means life, and *veda* means knowledge. Ayurveda is the science of living. As a complete system that treats each person as an individual, ayurveda is perfectly customized for you, and you can learn to analyze your personality type, body type, and lifestyle. Full of common sense, it equips you to take responsibility for your own well-being. Good health really is our natural state, but sometimes we block it. Ayurveda uses lifestyle, diet, and herbs to help remove such blocks and let you be the best *you* you can possibly be. This book is not intended as a substitute for medical advice. However, as an adjunct to your doctor's care, it offers both a complete holistic view of your health and helpful tools that you can use to rebalance your body, mind, and spirit.

A few hours of reading *The Ayurvedic Year* will give you both the basic knowledge you need to understand yourself better, and the tools you require to reharmonize body, mind, and spirit. With your new understanding, it will seem perfectly obvious and natural to make a few rebalancing lifestyle alterations.

Applying the principles of ayurveda will help you trust yourself to grow. You'll realize that many answers can be found within yourself. You know your body better than anyone—after all, you've had it all your life! Seeking information and advice from professionals or other sources is helpful, but the answers must make sense to you on an intuitive level. Even without an ayurvedic doctor on hand, you can use your powers of self-referral. Consider recent changes in your life, your lifestyle, the season, the weather, and your mental and physical state to develop an intuitive understanding of yourself and then make appropriate dietary or lifestyle alterations to head off an illness before it takes hold. In our outward-looking society with our outward-looking senses, we tend to look without. But often the key is within. Develop your ability to look within using ayurveda.

With ayurveda, your confidence will develop as you practice self-referral. Open yourself up to the answers that come from inside.

the ayurvedic toolbox

Ayurveda empowers you to not only diagnose, but correct imbalances in your life. This book teaches you about your constitutional type, which ayurveda calls your *dosha*. Use the quiz on pages 18–21 to understand your own special mix, then read about each dosha at the beginning of parts 2, 3, and 4.

Ayurveda tells us the base for good health is rooted in everyday diet and lifestyle. Part 1 gives tips on what to eat, how to eat, and how much to eat for optimal health. It concludes with suggestions for bringing more balance into your daily life.

In the chapters dedicated to each dosha, contributions to good health are outlined in detail. You will learn to improve aspects of your well-being that have been neglected, whether they be a dietary excess or deficiency, persistent negative thoughts, or chronic overwork. Beneficial foods and menus are suggested in each dosha section, and part 2 includes a section on weight management.

Information suitable to each dosha type is given on detoxification, massage, aromatherapy, color therapy, yoga postures, breathing exercises, visualization, and meditation. As your understanding of the doshas grows, just what is best for you will become more and more apparent. As you will find yourself to be a mix of all three doshas, you'll have the skills to make intuitive adjustments where necessary.

the benefits of yoga

A yoga sequence has been created for each dosha. The poses have been chosen to counter the weaknesses of each dosha and better balance the whole system. It is important to keep in mind that any yoga pose done in an appropriate way can help any dosha type.

❶ Regularity is the key. A daily twenty-minute yoga session is more life enhancing than a ninety-minute session once a week.

❷ Always practice yoga on an empty stomach. Let three or four hours pass after a large meal, and two hours after a snack.

❸ Wear comfortable, non-restrictive clothing. A yoga mat provides a hygienic, cushioned, non-slip surface.

❹ Pain in the joints or muscles might lead to injury, so always check your alignment in the position. As you practice, find your deepest point of stretch, while it still feels comfortable. Don't push your body forcefully past this point.

❺ Stay mentally present. If you sense your mind has wandered off, gently bring it back to concentrate on what you are doing. Absorb yourself in your breath and body sensations.

Cautions

If you are suffering from a health condition or have an injury, seek guidance from an experienced yoga teacher. If you are running a temperature, don't practice the postures or breathing exercises. Women should avoid inverted positions like Sarvangasana (Shoulder stand, pages 114–15), and Halasana (Plow Pose, pages 116–17) during menstruation. Instead practice restorative poses like supported Janu Shirshasana (Seated Head-to-Knee, pages 238–39), Supta Baddha Konasana (Reclining Bound Angle Pose, pages 178-79), Savasana (Corpse Pose, pages 244–45), and Savasana II (Breathing Easy Position, pages 180-81), which suit all doshas. Countless women have enjoyed the benefits of yoga during their pregnancies, but the first trimester of pregnancy is not a good time to start yoga. As many poses need modification during pregnancy, it's best to attend specialized classes during the second and third trimesters.

Cautionary guidelines are given throughout the yoga practice pages in each dosha section.

part I

the three doshas

Each of us is a special, unique human being. Just as no one is composed of just one dosha—we are born with all three elements within—no two people have the same Vata-Pitta-Kapha balance.

the three

"Ayurveda is the science of living."

doshas

contents:

introducing the doshas

Each person is made up of their own special mix of the three fundamental energies, or doshas. Although we can't see them, the three doshas are responsible for all processes of the mind and body. They affect our physical makeup and our mental and emotional qualities. Like the foundations of a building, these underlying forces determine who we are, what we like to eat, how thirsty we get, and how much sleep we need. They influence our reactions to stress and our predisposition to illness. They even affect how compassionate, relaxed, or talkative we are.

prakriti

From the moment of conception, each person has a unique blend of the three doshas. This underlying constitutional type, which makes up the essential part of our being, is known as *prakriti*. Prakriti is the basic constitution and tendencies we are born with. Each individual's prakriti, just like his or her fingerprints, is unlike anyone else's.

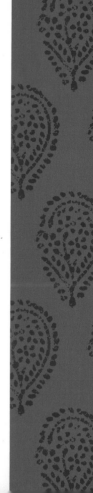

vrikriti

Superimposed on our underlaying prakriti is the way we lead our lives. Life is a never-ending flow of fluctuating factors. In fact, as we move through life, change is the only thing that doesn't change. We are constantly nudged to grow, alter, and adapt as we are confronted by the ongoing alteration of conditions around us. This process called life really keeps us on our toes, and although the underlying constitution we were born with doesn't alter, the expressions of it do. Our special mix of the three doshas changes from minute to minute, day to day, and season to season. The doshas influence how we eat, drink, sleep, work, play, exercise, and express ourselves. Climate, season, time of day, and stage of life all have an effect, too. This day-to-day variance, like a layer superimposed on the prakriti, is called *vrikriti*. Vrikriti refers to the temporary states of flux in the doshas.

identifying the doshas

❶ Vata, the moving force, expresses itself in kinetic energy. It takes care of all motion in the body and mind. It moves food through the digestive system and is involved in nerve conduction, blood circulation, and the skeletal and reproductive systems. It is active in the flow of thoughts and emotions. Vata has qualities of airiness, dryness, cold, and motion.

❷ Pitta, the transformative force, gives the power of transformation. It has moist, sharp, and hot qualities. Pitta is most active in the digestive system, giving us the ability to change nutrients into energy. Pitta is hot and fiery. It gives a person determination and focus.

❸ Kapha, the binding force, provides structure. It has earthy, watery, oily, and cold qualities. Kapha charges us with the potential energy needed to maintain the entire system. Kapha gives weight and stability to the organism. It oversees lubrication, including gastric juices and fluids in the joints.

working together

All doshas are active at all times but in varying degrees—this is why different symptoms and behaviors manifest. The digestive system offers a good example of how the doshas work together. The mobile element Vata is involved in chewing the food to start the process of breaking it down. The Kapha secretions of the salivary enzymes and gastric juices complete the job. The Kapha force also lubricates the food so it passes easily from mouth to stomach. As a catalyst, Pitta supplies digestive fire so the food can be broken down by enzymes and made ready for absorption. The food moves to the small intestine (a Vata organ), where it is absorbed and transformed into energy (a Pitta force). The nutrients are carried around the blood (Pitta) for delivery to the cells that need them (Vata). Any food not absorbed is transported through the colon for excretion (a Vata action).

Life is a dynamic interchange among the three doshas. Any alteration in one affects both of the others. Once you begin to understand the actions and interactions of the doshas, you will gain the knowledge and develop the intuition you need to bring yourself back into balance before you stray too far from your innate state of equilibrium.

assessing your doshas

Each cell in the body is created with a blend of Vata, Pitta, and Kapha, and so each of us is a mix of all three doshas. Use this test to assess your unique dosha blend. Consider each statement, and assign the number that is most appropriate beside each one (0, 2, or 4). Total the numbers at the bottom of each column and then add them together to establish your score for each dosha.

vata	never applies (0)	sometimes applies (2)	often applies (4)
My skin is dry. I can't seem to moisturize enough.			
I'm slim and can eat whatever I want without putting on weight.			
My digestion feels irregular: Sometimes I'm ravenous; sometimes I have no appetite.			
I learn new things easily, but my long-term memory isn't great.			
I am creative and enthusiastic.			
I give out so much energy that sometimes I need to rest up to recover.			
My energy levels fluctuate a lot.			
I dislike the cold, be it in weather, food, or drinks.			
My moods change easily.			
Stress makes me feel fearful and insecure.			
Subtotal score:			

pitta	never applies (0)	sometimes applies (2)	often applies (4)
I am of medium build and have a well-balanced shape.			
When I get indigestion, it tends to manifest as burning sensations.			
I love iced drinks, ice cream, and other cold foods.			
I have a large appetite and digest food very quickly.			
My mind is generally well-focused and alert.			
People consider me passionate, confident, and courageous.			
I don't like heat much: It tires me, and I sweat easily.			
I tend to be impatient, and sometimes anger easily.			
I am determined, critical, and stubborn.			
I'm rarely daunted by a challenge.			

Subtotal score:

Now that you know your scores for Vata and Pitta, continue the assessment on the next page and then calculate your final score. You can analyze your result with the advice given on page 21.

TO READ ABOUT EACH DOSHA IN DETAIL, TURN TO THE FOLLOWING PAGES:
kapha PART 2, PAGES 65-127, **pitta** PART 3, PAGES 129-191, **vata** PART 4, PAGES 193-253.

kapha	never applies (0)	sometimes applies (2)	often applies (4)
I have a solid build. As a baby, I was big boned.			
My digestion is slow, and I feel heavy after eating.			
I gain weight easily and am slow to lose it.			
I am patient and even tempered.			
I'm able to remain calm and unruffled under stress.			
I feel I'm slower than others to grasp new concepts.			
Once I really learn something, I never forget it.			
Once I get going, I have loads of stamina, but I'm not a high-energy person.			
I have a caring, compassionate nature.			
I don't like humidity and dampness, but I'm fine in very hot or very cold conditions.			
Subtotal score:			

Now add up each of your three dosha sub-totals, and insert the totals in the boxes below.

Total scores:

Vata		Pitta		Kapha	

analyzing your results

❶ Your highest scores reveal your most active doshas; the lower scores, your least active. Most people have one less-active and two more-active doshas.

❷ If two of your dosha scores are relatively close, you are bidoshic, with two predominant doshas. These doshas may express themselves at alternating moments or may work at the same time, side by side. How close your scores are gives you a clue to how much attention to pay through the changing seasons to keeping each dosha in balance, as each dosha holds different influences in each season.

❸ If your three scores are all similar, have a friend help you go over the questions. Uncertainty is a sign of Vata, so lean toward this dosha if you are unsure about your answers. A few rare people are tridoshic, manifesting all three doshas in similar amounts. If you are tridoshic, you have been given a great start toward good balance, and the opportunity to be healthy, long-lived, and emotionally stable. On the other hand, once the three doshas get out of balance, it's more difficult to reharmonize them: Rather than concentrating on one dosha first and then a second, three points of focus call simultaneously for attention.

finding a healthy balance

Our doshas are the lenses through which we view the world. As the old saying goes, "It takes all kinds," and there are as many variations of "normal" as there are people on the earth. Vata types tend to believe that it's normal to be always on the move and that to be any other way is just odd. For forward-looking Pitta types, strong determination and ambition are part of the usual mode of existence, and they find someone who lacks those qualities difficult to understand. Kaphas can experience lovely serenity and contentment by staying right where they are. Taking things slow and steady is normal for them, so they might not understand the ambition of Pittas or the way Vatas are forever coming up with new projects.

Just where a healthy balance lies is different for each person. Each dosha achieves its own beauty when it takes advantage of its particular qualities and finds a good balance with the others. While the Pitta traits of ambition and drive are considered admirable in our society, they are not so attractive when they turn into ruthlessness and hardness because of a lack of Kapha compassion and serenity. In conversation, Vata types are vivacious, quick-witted, and charming, but without the caring open-heartedness of Kapha, gossipy jokes can turn ugly. Although brimming with new ideas, a Vata may never turn a single one into reality without some of

the stability of Kapha or the drive of Pitta. Kapha, with its solid foundation, risks never getting started without some of Vata's enthusiasm or Pitta's determination.

Managing your life is like running your own business. To be successful, you need Vata to think up and champion ideas born of creativity and enthusiasm. The ambition, drive, and determination of Pitta are needed to see the ideas through to completion. And the steady, reliable, sustaining force of Kapha is essential, since it doesn't mind the routine work that must be done, and it has the stamina to keep things going when Pitta and Vata have tired.

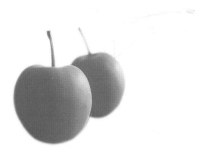

understanding others

A basic understanding of the doshas allows your compassion toward others to grow. When a Vata finds out that her couch-potato house companion is predominantly Kapha, she can understand why he chooses to stay in every night. When a Pitta realizes that his colleague is strongly Vata, it's easier for him to understand why she lacks the follow-through to close a deal. When a Kapha grasps that her husband has hardly any Kapha, it's easier for her to accept his lack of patience in listening to her troubles.

There is beauty in each dosha when it finds its healthy state. Currently, western society considers a slim, Vata-type super-model body most desirable; in the past, the rounder Kapha build of Sophia Loren types was more popular. People go under the knife for a symmetrical, even-featured Pitta face. But real beauty is to be found in the integral harmony within each dosha. Nature continually moves in the direction of harmonious balance— nothing is sustainable without it—so release yourself from the artificial constraints of Hollywood and advertising, and find contentment in the true beauty of your own balance.

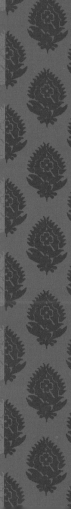

getting to know yourself

Understanding your special dosha mix is a fantastic tool in getting to know yourself better. Self-knowledge fosters self-acceptance. Knowledge of the doshas helps you identify and appreciate your positive traits and take responsibility for your less desirable ones. While you reharmonize body and mind with the tools of ayurveda, stay patient and tolerant. Send compassion to yourself even when you think you've failed. Too often, self-criticism becomes incredibly self-destructive. We would never dream of applying the unkind and destructive comments, attitudes, and expectations of our inner monologues to another person. Yet such negative self-judgments can be relentless.

Accepting and appreciating positive attributes is cause for celebration. Inevitably, you will have traits you don't welcome, but often these can be altered or minimized with lifestyle changes that better balance your doshic mix. Accepting your fundamental nature gives you a realistic base from which to work and supports you as you grow. The aim is not to create a new you but to remain true to yourself as you become the best possible you.

true health

We should not aim merely to be symptom free. True health is much more than the standard medical definition of "an absence of disease"; it demands a high level of vitality in your whole mind, body, and spirit. True health gives you the vibrant energy you need to perform your daily and lifelong tasks effectively and joyfully.

Think back to a time when you were truly happy. You had an abundance of energy and enthusiasm for every task, you slept well, and you laughed often. Your life had direction—perhaps you were studying a subject you enjoyed, found satisfaction in raising your family, or felt very fulfilled in your work. You had a clear spiritual base and felt a strong sense of community with friends and others that you may have helped who were in need. Think back. Did you notice that you didn't catch the flu that was going around, or that a chronic ailment bothered you less? Just as your mind is more tranquil when your body is healthy, your body is stronger when you are happy.

Does this happy state seem unrealistic now? Even in the most adverse situation, or with a very serious health condition, it is possible to bring better balance into your life. Use the tools of ayurveda to go for glowing good health.

"True health is an abundance of energy and enthusiasm, a spring in your step, and the capacity to laugh out loud."

five dimensions of health

Ayurveda recognizes five dimensions of subtle anatomy that make up each person. These dimensions are *koshas*, meaning "sheaths." True health occurs when each sheath functions well. The first sheath is the physical body. The second is the vital force, composed of prana, the essential energy in everything alive. The third sheath is our mental state—thoughts and feelings. The fourth kosha, the sheath of wisdom, deals with how we intuit and understand everything around us. Finally, the fifth sheath relates to our spiritual selves. Meditation works on this level, helping us transcend physical or mental discomfort and giving us a sense of connection with a protective, nurturing force larger than ourselves.

Although only the first sheath is visible, the five koshas have a huge effect on health. Since no one thing is independent of another, an imbalance in a single sheath filters through to manifest symptoms in others. In fact, the more subtle the sheath, the more influence it has. Prana is more subtle than the dense physical body, so blockage or stagnation of prana causes symptoms in the physical body. A blockage in the mind affects the vital force as well as the physical body. Similarly, a positive mind benefits the physical body—a placebo sugar pill is efficient medicine for the body, at least in the short term, because of the healing power of positive thought.

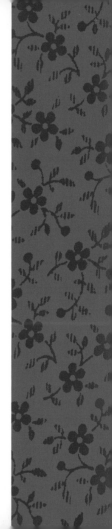

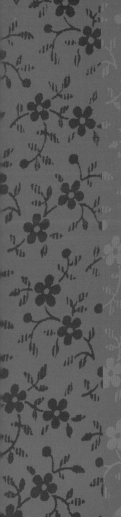

you are more than your illness

With chronic disease, it's easy to define yourself by your condition, when in reality you are much more than any illness. Why not replace "I am diabetic" with "I am a wonderful, whole person with high blood sugar levels"? Or swap "I am asthmatic" for "I am a calm, loving person with a breathing disorder"? Harmony can be found even in a state of serious illness if you view yourself on more than just a physical level. Indeed, it is possible to be healthy on many levels yet carry an illness on another. Keeping the positive in mind helps you maintain a strong sense of self, connected to a greater healing force—a wonderful asset when you are confronted by pain, cancer, heart disease, or other ailments.

whole health

"You are what you eat," and while we are literally composed of what we eat, we are much more than that. We are also what we think. Every year almost all of the body's cells are replaced. Think of cells being created in moments of sadness, depression, or anger. If you believe "heart disease runs in my family," cells are created with this energy within them. The belief affects your health. It feels better to think of cells being created with positive energy when you feel calm, content, and full of hope for the future.

modern medicine
and ayurveda

The word *health* in old English is linked to the word *whole*. Health can be defined as the experience of wholeness—feeling integrated and being at one with yourself. Unfortunately, for some health conditions, modern medicine is better at symptom control than lasting cure. Rather than searching to alleviate the cause of the condition (which can be in any kosha and may be a nutrient deficiency, work-related stress, or a broken heart), conventional medicine sometimes zeros in on just treating the symptoms (bleeding gums, insomnia, or depression).

Ayurveda takes into account all the layers that make up a person. Modern medicine, in contrast, splits us into smaller parts. You consult an ear, nose, and throat specialist for enlarged tonsils, an endocrinologist for premenstrual syndrome, a cardiologist for heart palpitations. Modern medicine is wonderfully helpful, particularly in the acute stages of disease, but for some conditions it can often only temporarily relieve symptoms or slow their progression. Alternative medicine may offer greater relief, in providing greater awareness of how to assess and rebalance your personal well-being.

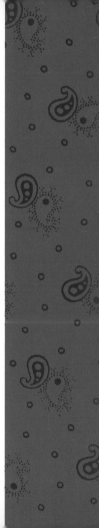

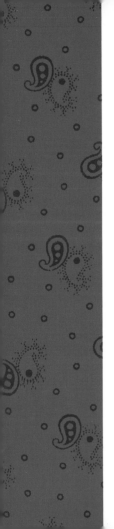

wake up to your symptoms

A healthy diet, a healthy lifestyle, and a positive outlook preserve health and help prevent major killers, such as cancer and heart disease. But if you have already developed a disease, reframe your attitude to the inconvenient symptoms of your lack of ease. Discomfort is a helpful wake-up call. It sounds obvious, but pain is painful. We naturally move away from it. Take the opportunity to move toward personal growth. Consider whether you are just masking your pain with anti-inflammatories, surgery, and suppressive treatments. Too often we strap up a twisted ankle and soldier on, ignoring a clear signal to rest. Pain is your body asking you to listen. It starts by whispering; if you ignore it, it might have to shout. Use ayurveda to help you recognize symptoms at an early stage, when they are more easily treated. Ayurveda can help undo past wrongs, too. Your body is a forest. If it was once full of tall, healthy trees yet now feels deforested, ayurveda gives you the knowledge and tools to help the trees regrow. Reconnect with your inner harmony and flourish.

six stages of disease

Ayurveda recognizes six levels of disease. The sooner you notice an imbalance forming, the sooner you can counter it. The earlier you head off the imbalance, the easier and gentler the treatment will be. Ayurvedic medicine can even recognize your potential to develop disease later in life so that you can take preventive measures now.

Disease is caused by an imbalance of the doshas. It can creep up slowly over time or, if the cause is sudden, can come on rapidly. The ayurvedic approach to illness recognizes six stages of the onset of disease. The initial stage is caused when a certain dosha increases at a faster rate than the body can deal with or manage to release. The second phase is characterized by a feeling of unease, and this nearly always manifests first in the mind. The mind is less comfortable and less alert than usual; you sense that something is not quite right. Possible early physical symptoms include indigestion.

Western medicine, in the absence of concrete symptoms, cannot make a diagnosis at this time and so can do little to help. There are few conventional options for someone who has back pain when an x-ray shows no irregularities or feels tired when blood tests find no problems. Happily, ayurvedic medicine makes it possible for you to take precautions early on.

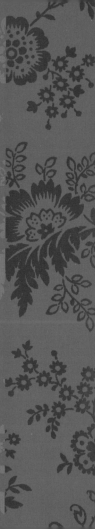

When an imbalance persists through stages one and two, small clues may appear in other tissues as the imbalance spreads through the system in stage three. Laboratory tests still may not show irregularities. By stage four, symptoms will be clear enough to lead to a diagnosis by medical practitioners. The situation worsens through stage five. By stage six, the body system is clearly weakened. Even if the doshic imbalance is treated and symptoms alleviated, the body system will be weak and the imbalance may have spread to other areas. For permanent healing, you must address the root cause of your condition rather than mere symptoms.

ayurvedic diagnosis

An ayurvedic doctor observes the physical appearance and other characteristics of a patient, including body type, coloring, features, gait, skin type, posture, and voice. These give clues to the state of the doshas and their tendencies toward derangement. The practitioner takes a detailed case history, examines the tongue for signs of coating, and feels the pulses (doshic imbalance is evident in the pulses at a very early stage). A diagnosis of the state of the doshas is then made, and recommendations are given on how to balance them.

your tendencies

When you have any sort of imbalance—physical, energetic, mental, or emotional—stress tends to manifest in the weakest organ of your physical body. Some people easily pick up colds or battle a seemingly constant sniffle. Others may tend to have flare-ups of a skin condition, insomnia, asthma attacks, constipation, or depression.

You probably already know that part of your body is weaker than the rest and manifests symptoms most readily. Use the ayurvedic tools of diet, lifestyle, and mindset to do something about it. Get to know your temperament, physical requirements, emotional needs, desires, aims, ambitions, actions, and reactions to stimuli.

the effects of stress

You may have noticed that when you are faced with a small amount of stress, such as that caused by a deadline, you become more efficient. The adrenal glands produce more adrenaline and, up to a certain point, some stress is useful. However, when the stress is too great, the system becomes fatigued. After months or years of unrelenting stressful conditions, the adrenal glands begin to fail. In becoming less efficient they produce less adrenaline. The system can no longer keep up, and exhaustion sets in. The only answer is to rest and nurture yourself back to health, however long it takes.

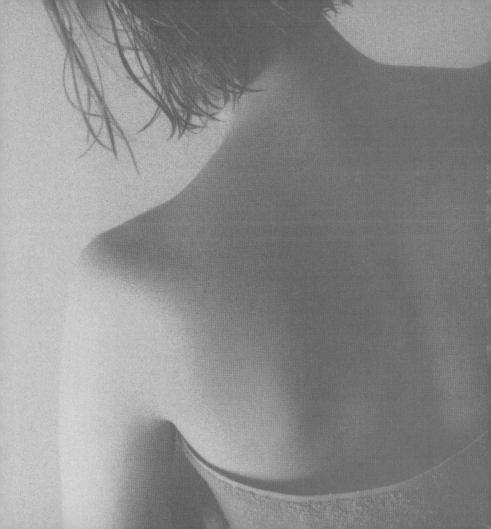

ayurvedic treatments

In general, ayurvedic treatments are more natural and, therefore, less harmful than the treatments of western allopathic medicine. Ayurveda uses diet and lifestyle as initial treatments, saving herbal therapy for more firmly entrenched conditions. By emphasizing self-awareness, rest, activity, diet, and thoughts, ayurveda allows you to be proactive in your healing. Learning how to monitor and improve your health with ayurveda equips you well for life.

Although this book does not attempt to replace conventional medical care, it does give you the tools you need to keep tabs on your health yourself. Taking charge of your health rather than having to rely solely on a doctor's observations and prescriptions is wonderfully empowering. You are a vital and vibrant being and are meant to realize your true potential. Throughout life, knowledge of ayurveda supports you as you do the best you can to meet life's challenges and earn its rewards.

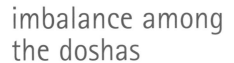

imbalance among the doshas

According to ayurveda, disease occurs when the balance of the three doshas is disturbed. The cause may be a single factor or a mix of many: Hereditary, dietary, environmental, and emotional factors; climate; lack of rest; or improper diet. While the doshas don't work in isolation, each dosha does have an affinity with certain organs, symptoms, and types of diseases, as the charts on the next few pages show.

Should a single dosha increase, it tends to decrease the other two, and you should work on rebalancing the aggravated dosha by using the ideas found in the relevant parts of this book:

• Kapha (Part 2, pages 65-127)
• Pitta (Part 3, pages 129-91)
• Vata (Part 4, pages 193-253).

Should two or all three doshas manifest symptoms, begin by balancing the most aggravated one, or the one that is strongest in your constitution. If you cannot decide which dosha is most aggravated, work first on Vata; as the mobile force, it has a strong sway on the other doshas.

Ayurveda becomes easy to understand and apply once you have a clear vision of each dosha. Ayurveda tells us that one quality will be decreased by its opposite. When you have overworked, the key is to rest. When physical inactivity has let the mind become sluggish, increased movement stimulates body and mind to bring about balance. Eating dry foods counterbalances Kapha's moistness but increases Vata. When increased, Vata makes the system dry and the mind unsettled: Counter with an oil massage or the warm, calming humidity of a long bath. A long, hot bath, like the hot summer season, increases Pitta, which can be balanced by cooler environments.

Use the charts on pages 40-41 to pinpoint doshic imbalances that may be causing your health problems and to find ways to reharmonize your system.

analyzing your excess doshas

The charts that follow will help you examine the nature of your doshic imbalance. By considering the qualities listed, you can identify how your pain might relate to Vata, Pitta, and Kapha. Step back from the name of your disease and examine your condition from a fresh perspective. Consider the nature of the symptoms, the quality of the pains, the location of the condition, and how the condition manifests in the mind.

self-diagnosis tips
• Often, the first symptom of an aggravated dosha appears at its seat *(see page 41)*. The greater the severity of the symptom, the greater the aggravation will be.
• You may notice a tendency toward one dosha and, at certain times, flare-ups caused by another dosha.
• Discover your tendencies *(see pages 34–35)*: It's helpful to work out where your weaker areas are, and to observe these first to gain clues to the state of your doshas.

timing and qualities
of symptoms

Each dosha rules a time of day, a season, and a stage of life. When making a self-diagnosis, note what time of the day and the year the symptoms began, and trace when the symptoms worsen.

For more in-depth information about the characteristics of eash dosha, see Kapha, pages 68–73; Pitta, pages 132–36; and Vata, pages 196–201.

dosha	Vata	Pitta	Kapha
times of the day	before dawn through the early morning and late afternoon through the early evening	the two or three hours before and after midnight	mornings from 7 to 10 am and evenings from 6 to 10 pm
seasons	fall and early winter	late spring and early summer	winter and early spring
stages of life	old age	early adulthood to gradual old age	birth to adolescence

Look for the following qualities and affinities of each dosha when assessing the symptoms of your health problems.

dosha	Vata	Pitta	Kapha
seat in the body	Colon	Small intestine	Stomach
other affinities	Lower back, skin, nervous system, pelvis, thighs, bones, ears, and skin	Stomach, liver, spleen, gall bladder, endocrine glands, blood, and sweat	Lungs, mucous membranes, lymphatic system, joints, lubrication via body secretions
main symptom	Pain	Inflammation	Fluid symptoms, such as pus or mucus
general nature of symptoms	Transient, changeable symptoms. Dry conditions, such as dehydration, constipation, dry eczema; dry skin, hair, brittle nails. Colds. Conditions of increased movement, such as faster heartbeats, cramps, prolapses, insomnia, and diarrhea	Hot conditions, such as fevers, inflammations, irritations, hot flushes, sunburn, rashes, acne, and sweating. Symptoms characterized by burning, such as hyperacidity, fever, inflammation, ulceration. Bleeding disorders, jaundice	Oily, dense, or heavy symptoms, such as congestion of the nose or lungs, fluid retention, or discharges. Lethargic conditions of decreased tone, obesity, enlarged organs, or tumors. Kaphas tend toward asthma, high cholesterol levels, pallor, mental dullness
types of pains	Radiating, shifting, shooting, fluctuating, or pulsating pains	Sharp, piercing, burning, penetrating, intense pains or flushes	Heavy, deep, aching, or throbbing mild pains
mental and emotional symptoms	Confusion, mental chaos, fear, anxiety, memory loss, dizziness	Irritation, mood swings, anger, frustration, jealousy, and being argumentative or critical	Depression, sluggishness, listlessness, and excessive sleep

ayurveda through the seasons

In Indian thought, the mind and spirit cannot be separated from the body, giving rise to the concept of the *bodymind*, a word recognizing the intrinsic links between mind, body, and spirit. Ayurveda teaches us to respect the effects of changing times of day and seasons on the bodymind. Working with the seasons leads to better health: Any imbalance, whether it manifests as fatigue, cancer, heart disease, or itchy skin, stands to be corrected. Since the seasons are a force of great sustenance, it makes sense to align ourselves with them. It's so natural to clean out after Kapha winter that we have coined a phrase for it: Spring cleaning. It's so natural to try to stay cool during Pitta midday heat that many hot countries have developed the siesta.

Thanks to new cultivation, transportation, and exportation methods, most seasonal foods are now available in North America year-round, separating us from nature. Ayurveda emphasizes how it is best to eat locally grown, seasonal foods that connect us to our regions. In this technological age, we need to remind ourselves how to live naturally to rediscover an inner trust that intuits what we need to stay healthy. Then, mind, spirit, and body will be healthy.

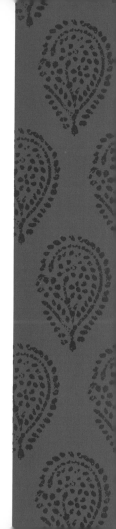

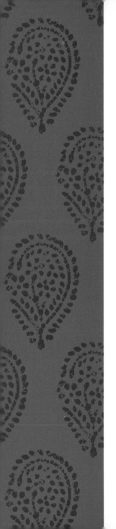

seasonal living

The seasons, according to ayurveda, are different in different regions of the world. Rather than using set calendar dates to determine when you should make seasonal changes in your lifestyle, consider the climate of your region, keeping in mind that even in the same place, the timing of the seasons varies from year to year. In India and other tropical countries, each year may have six seasons because of the monsoon. European cities such as London have four seasons. From the ayurvedic viewpoint, more temperate zones around the world, for example Mexico, may be divided into three seasons. Any change in the weather increases or decreases each dosha.

Because of the continual flux of nature, any dosha can increase regardless of season. Even in midsummer, a chilly, dry spell increases Vata and decreases Pitta. Humid overcast weather increases Kapha and decreases Vata, even if it is warm. A warmer period in winter causes Pitta to increase and Kapha and Vata to decrease. Consider where you live and how clearly demarcated the seasons are to understand how much to alter your lifestyle through the year. When you move between regions, you may notice a "season lag." While jet lag might last a few days, the body can take longer to adjust to a sudden change in season.

[43]

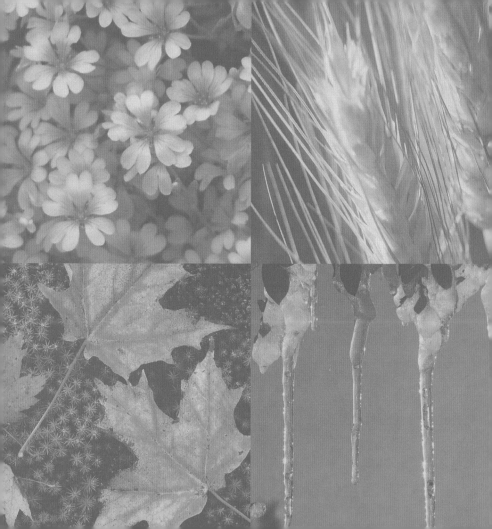

changing with the seasons

Ayurveda teaches daily and seasonal compensatory mechanisms to help you maintain health at all times. Should you fall ill, purification of the system is helpful. When you are healthy, a daily routine (see pages 60-63) augments health and rejuvenates. Regardless of the season, keep to your daily routine and adapt your diet and lifestyle to the changing year. When you maintain regular habits throughout the seasons, you are less prone to change-of-season illness.

When you fail to compensate for changes in the seasons or stages of life, imbalances arise. The junctions between seasons are common times to fall ill—many people catch a cold when the weather turns warm after winter, for instance. If you hibernate like a sleepy bear during winter, reducing your activity level and eating heavy foods with high dairy and fat content, your system starts to overload. By the time spring arrives, your body wants to clean out all that Kapha build-up, and a cold, hay fever, or wet cough—signs of excess Kapha—develops. When the seasons change, take a moment to be still, recenter, and detoxify. These are natural times to cleanse the bodymind using the techniques set out for each dosha.

examining your health condition

Ayurveda does not place great emphasis on naming each disease. Instead, it focuses on the qualities of each disease.

Looking holistically at the body, you will probably find that several seemingly unrelated symptoms are linked to a single imbalance. Once you find the cause, it's easier and, of course, more effective to target one imbalance than several symptoms. Ayurveda doesn't depend on the randomized, double-blind laboratory tests of modern science. It takes advantage of the wealth of knowledge of the ancients—the empirical learning of 5000 years of practice and observation. Here is how ayurveda understands some of the common ailments of the modern world.

indigestion

It is vital to digest well in order to give all body systems the best possible chance to be healthy. If digestion is poor, food is not properly broken down and nutrients are less easily absorbed. This affects repair and renewal of the cells of the body. Indigestion tends to manifest very early in any condition and is often the first sign of imbalance in the body.

Each dosha experiences indigestion as follows:

• Vata, with its erratic nature, makes digestion unpredictable. Digestion that is previously fine will suddenly change for no apparent reason. Vata tends toward constipation, and even when the diet remains constant, constipation may alternate with loose bowels. The appetite may change and the tongue be alternately coated and clear. (A coated tongue is a sign of toxins, *ama*.) The seat of Vata is the colon, and flatulence, a sign of Vata's mobile elements of air and ether, manifests here. An out-of-balance Vata feels the cold, craves hot food and drinks, and has increased anxiety, too.

• When fiery Pitta arises in the digestive system, it craves cold food and drinks to balance it. Burning symptoms may occur in the digestive system, and hyperacidity leads to heartburn or ulceration. The mouth may develop a sour taste. Pittas naturally tend toward loose bowels, so diarrhea may result from aggravated Pitta. The seat of Pitta is the small intestine, and food may pass through the intestines so quickly that nutrients can't be properly extracted. Bouts of Pitta anger may also manifest.

• Kapha causes the digestive system to feel full and heavy. Symptoms may manifest first in the seat of Kapha, the stomach. Digestion will be slow, so food tends to sit around for too long. The liquid element of Kapha may cause the mouth to water. In an effort to achieve balance, Kapha craves bitter and astringent foods. Mental lethargy sets in.

coughs and colds

The symptoms of the common cold also vary depending on which dosha is most active during the season you catch a cold.

• A dry cough with little mucus points to excessive Vata.

• Excess Pitta is signaled by hot symptoms, such as a raw throat. Green phlegm is another sign of Pitta.

• Heavy congestion and a cough with plenty of phlegm and a dulled mind point to Kapha.

menstrual complaints

It's helpful to analyze the symptoms of menstrual dysfunction through the doshas.

• Erratic Vata produces irregular cycles. The blood is dark or clotted, and spotting may occur. During the flow, or before it begins, there tends to be constipation, and this may alternate with loose stools. Vata produces cramps and pain. The airy element of Vata can give you a feeling of ungroundedness. Insomnia, mood swings, and anxiety can be part of the Vata premenstrual syndrome.

• The Pitta cycle is regular and may be short. Bleeding tends to be longer and heavy, and the blood is bright red or may have a black tinge. Cramps may be present but are not as strong as Vata's, and there can be loose stools. Pittas have food and sugar cravings and may feel hot, flushed, and touchy. Symptoms can show in the skin, and acne often flares up around the period.

• The Kapha cycle is regular and flow is average. Kapha tends toward fluid retention. Swelling of the breasts, abdominal bloating, and generalized edema are common. During the period, Kapha feels stiff in the bones and joints, and slow and lethargic in body and mind.

the importance of diet

The importance of a healthful diet must never be underestimated—it is the underlying support of good health, and if eating patterns are harmful, other treatments have trouble achieving a lasting cure. According to an Indian proverb, "You do not need medicine if your diet is right, and it is not medicine that you need if your diet is wrong." Ayurveda teaches you how to overcome disease with correct eating.

Unfortunately, the self-referral mechanism becomes damaged when tastebuds, fed on a diet of sugary drinks and fast food, are corrupted from a young age and lose their innate ability to judge which foods are appropriate. While western society has made notable advances in nutrition, these leaps of progress have caused us to lose touch with natural cycles. When we lived off the land, planting and reaping with the seasons, we ate foods appropriate for each time of year. With less international trade, we enjoyed local foods that automatically kept us in harmony with nature. Sweet cooling fruits ripened in time to counteract the Pitta heat of summer. Stored grains, slow-cooked stews, and salty preserved foods warmed us during the cold Kapha winter. On the one hand, hygiene has improved and nutrient deficiencies have decreased, but on the other, we would benefit from getting back in touch with

[50]

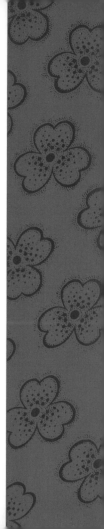

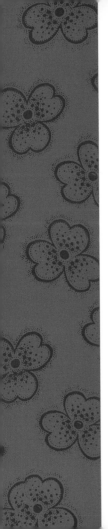

nature: Whole grains nourish better than refined foods; organic produce is more nutritious than foods containing artificial chemicals and pesticides. Our bodies are equipped to break down natural compounds that have been around for thousands of years; until we have evolved over future generations, we might have difficulty dealing with new compounds in additives and genetically modified crops.

conscious cooking

Ayurveda doesn't consider only the biological qualities of the nutrients in food; it also considers the energetic effects. When diet is used consciously to balance the bodymind, food becomes truly medicinal.

So if you can't cook, start learning! Ayurveda regards cooking, with its incredible power to keep us in good health, as an art form. Homemade food, cooked with love, nourishes the soul. Regularly taking the time to prepare food mindfully goes a long way toward keeping body and spirit healthy. By choosing different food combinations and cooking methods, you can fine-tune and correct the balance among the doshas. And since food should be pleasurable, the ayurvedic diet is not only therapeutic, it tastes delicious.

rasa—
the tastes of ayurveda

Food may be divided into six tastes, or *rasa*, and each rasa has links with the seasons. The rasa are a key to understanding the medicinal value of foods. Each taste influences the bodymind in a different way, and the effects continue even after digestion is completed. The six tastes also influence your consciousness. In the continuing dance to find a harmonious state, each taste is able to balance one or two doshas; conversely, one taste eaten in excess can aggravate a dosha.

Most foods are a combination of two or more tastes. By combining rich blends of spices and a variety of dishes at each meal, Indian cooking balances the six tastes well. Other cultures have also developed ways to balance the tastes in their cooking. Ideally, all six tastes should be present in every meal. When they are, a meal is enjoyably satisfying.

Churans are herb and spice blends that contain each of the six tastes in proportion. Since they are dosha balancing, you can easily personalize a meal by adding the appropriate churan. Vata, Kapha, and Pitta churan blends can be bought in ayurvedic and Indian grocery shops.

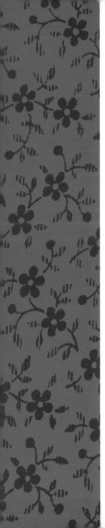

Tastes that increase each dosha

Vata	Pitta	Kapha
Bitter	Salty	Sweet
Astringent	Sour	Sour
Pungent	Pungent	Salty

Tastes that balance each dosha

Vata	Pitta	Kapha
Sour	Sweet	Pungent
Sweet	Bitter	Bitter
Salty	Astringent	Astringent

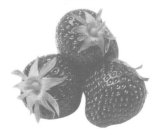

the six tastes

sweet: As well as naturally sweet foods, the sweet rasa includes grains, and vegetables that contain carbohydrates. Sweet rasa tends to slow digestion; it balances Vata and Pitta while increasing Kapha in the body. Too much results in symptoms such as obesity, diabetes, acidity, indigestion, and tumors. As winter is also the Kapha-increasing time, Kaphas do best to avoid the sweet taste then.

bitter: Bitterness brings freshness to a meal and mentally helps you see clearly. Radicchio, chicory, and most medicinal herbs are bitter. Olives, beer, tea, coffee, and natural chocolate have bitter qualities. The bitter rasa balances the heat of Pitta and the heaviness of Kapha and so can be used medicinally for these types in summer and winter, respectively. The bitter taste is Vata-increasing. Its season is fall and early winter.

sour: This zesty flavor is found in citrus fruit; sour fruit such as grapes, apples, or plums; tomatoes and some salad dressings; and aged or fermented foods, including cheese, vinegar, and pickles. The sour rasa promotes digestion, is good for the heart, and warms the body. Too much can cause burning sensations, loss of strength, irritation, dizziness, and premature aging. The sour taste relates to early fall; it balances excess Vata and increases Pitta.

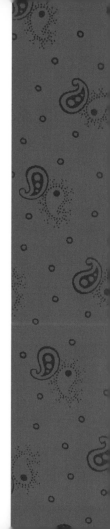

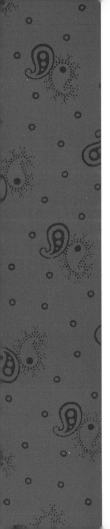

pungent: Garlic, onions, and hot spices such as chilies, peppers, cinnamon, and paprika are pungent. Summer is the time of the pungent rasa, which dries Kapha and can be used therapeutically during winter. In excess, pungent rasa can cause irritation and burning sensations (Pitta) or dizziness, dry mouth, increased thirst, and dry sexual secretions (Vata). Pungent foods are best limited during summer and fall. Mentally, pungent foods increase anger and aggression. The drying-out action can clear the mind.

salty: This flavor is found in soy sauce, seaweed, salted nuts and fries, and vegetable-based seasonings. Fast foods and canned foods are usually high in salt. Salt enhances digestion because it is warming. In excess, it causes water retention, and can lead to inflammatory conditions, skin and joint diseases, early baldness, and skin aging. Salt is Vata-balancing, so the best time to eat it is in fall.

astringent: This taste causes a puckering sensation on the tongue. Pomegranates, black tea, garbanzo beans, and unripe bananas are all astringent. The taste has a cooling effect, which moderates excess fire and slows digestion. In excess, it produces tremors, constipation, dryness of the body, numbness, and flatulence. Astringent foods balance Kapha and Pitta, so more of them may be eaten in winter and summer.

how to eat

Everything you eat affects the balance of your doshas, and so does the way in which food is prepared and eaten. As long as your regular food is wholesome, your body will tolerate the occasional splurge: Moderation in all things, including moderation.

general tips
• Ayurveda recommends cooked food. Raw food contains enzymes that assist the digestive system, and raw food has more vitamins than cooked food. However, cooked food is more easily digested, and the nutrients are assimilated more efficiently. Cereals, pulses, meats, and root vegetables are more easily digested when cooked, than if eaten raw. Many people with upset digestion, especially gain relief from an all-cooked diet.

• Whole foods beat refined foods. It's more natural to eat an orange than to drink orange juice or take vitamin C (which lacks everything an orange offers, including its sustaining life force).

• Low-chemical foods are better than those containing preservatives, emulsifiers, insecticides, or hormones. Choose fresh, seasonal, and organic ingredients.

• Eat ingredients that support your temperament and are appropriate to the climate. Vata and Kapha constitutions need warming foods. Also, Kapha, with its wet qualities, does best with dry foods. Pitta types need foods that cool.

• Limit your intake of water while eating. Drinking a lot of water with meals cools *agni*, the digestive fire.

• Don't eat too little or too much. Put both hands together, as if you were ready to have grain poured into them. This is a two-hand measure, or two *anjali*, your stomach's capacity at one sitting. It takes the stomach 20 minutes to tell the brain it's full. If, after eating two anjali, you feel like eating more, wait at least five minutes and see how you feel then. Leave one third of the stomach empty so that food can mix with digestive juices.

• Avoid snacking. Food takes three to four hours to leave the stomach. Don't eat the next meal until the last one has left your stomach. This lets the digestive system focus on processing food without disturbance. Kapha may do well on just two meals a day. Vata does better on four small ones.

eating for pleasure

How you eat is as important as what you eat. You have two nervous systems, the sympathetic and parasympathetic. The parasympathetic nervous system, the rest and repair system, is the one needed for digestion. When you are under stress, the sympathetic nervous system, involved in the adrenaline response, is activated and the parasympathetic nervous system is turned off. This decreases your digestive power, and food sits in your body longer. When food stays in the bowel too long, it starts to ferment and create gas. Harmful metabolites form, and toxins may be absorbed across the intestinal wall into the bloodstream, creating health problems.

mindful eating

Eating is a sensual experience. Make it pleasurable with background music, candles, and flowers. Share conversation with friends and family. Don't rush. Sit down and chew food properly, to help prevent the stomach and intestines having to work harder. As you eat, focus on your food and all of its colors, tastes, and textures. Splurge occasionally, and enjoy it. There is no point in feeling guilty or ashamed.

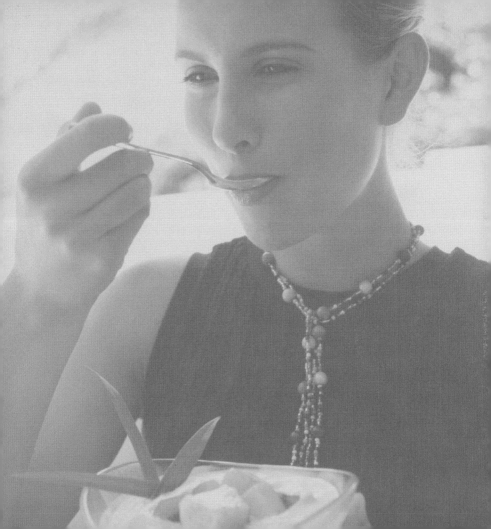

your daily routine

Imagine that your body is a garden. If you water it regularly, it flourishes. If you ignore it for weeks and then drown it, it may be so dry it can't accept the water it eventually receives. Adopting a regular daily routine is like watering your internal garden. A little time invested in your body pays dividends later. Start building good habits with one or two tips below, and add to them in time.

get enough sleep

Sleep enough to wake refreshed and ready for the day. Don't cheat your health with a constant sleep deficit or overtax your mind by making it perform in a haze of tiredness. However, if you are a Kapha type, don't use this as an excuse to oversleep.

write down your dreams

Dreams often communicate subconscious messages. If you think your dreams have special significance, jot them down on a notepad kept next to the bed and ponder their meaning later.

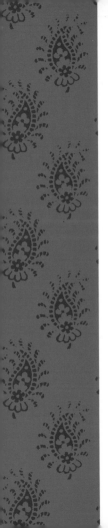

start the day with mental cleansing

Repeat an affirmation about your day ahead: "I feel
great!" "Today will be wonderful," or "I will be kind and
loving today." Then mentally connect the affirmation with
a small object such as a ring or a pebble that you can
carry all day. Each time you see or touch that special
object, repeat the affirmation.

exercise

Early morning is a Vata time, and as Vata is related to
movement it's a natural time for physical activity. Taking
an early morning walk or stretching for just five minutes
sets you up for the day.

brush your skin

Help eliminate toxins in your body by exfoliatng dead skin
cells. Brush dry skin with a natural-bristle body brush
before showering. Start from the extremities and use
short strokes, always moving toward the heart. Don't forget the soles of the feet and the palms of the hands. Keep
the strokes lighter on more sensitive areas, such as the
abdomen, and avoid the genitals and face.

practice yoga breathing

Correct breathing calms the mind and helps you start the day with the right attitude. With deep breathing, you tap into a new source of energy. *For Kapha, see pages 124–5, for Pitta, see pages 182–7, and for Vata, see pages 246–9.*

oil your skin

Oil massage improves the circulation of blood and lymph so that metabolic wastes can be removed. Kapha and Pitta types should do this once a week. If you are strongly Vata, oil your skin three times a week. For instructions, see page 222.

clean your tongue and teeth

After you have brushed your teeth, scrape your tongue twice from back to tip. This removes ama built up in the coating on the tongue, and mucus that may house bacteria. A special tongue scraper, a metal U-shaped device, is available in ayurvedic or Indian shops.

meditate

The benefits of meditation are far-reaching, and meditation is a wonderful, centering way to start the day. In the morning, the mind is calmer, more alert. In the evening, meditation can help you process the day's events.

hydrate
Squeeze half a lemon into a glass of warm water. Then rinse with pure water to stimulate the liver and cleanse the digestive system. Use a juicer to juice your favorite fruits and vegetables.

eat a healthy breakfast
The ideal diet differs from person to person. Choose a breakfast appropriate to your dosha—see Kapha, page 85; Pitta, page 150; and Vata, page 214.

invest in yourself
Think of something that would improve your quality of life, something to feed your soul and help you develop. Perhaps you could further your creativity with an art or dance course, take time out to talk with inspiring friends, or find a regular time for silence. You could volunteer to help others, quietly commune with nature, pursue further studies, or follow the guidelines in this book. When you have decided what you want to do, make a commitment to do it. Write it in your calendar, being realistic about the time you need, and don't let pressing matters erode the time away. Whether you settle on a couple of hours each weekend or 15 minutes a day, stick to your investment in yourself.

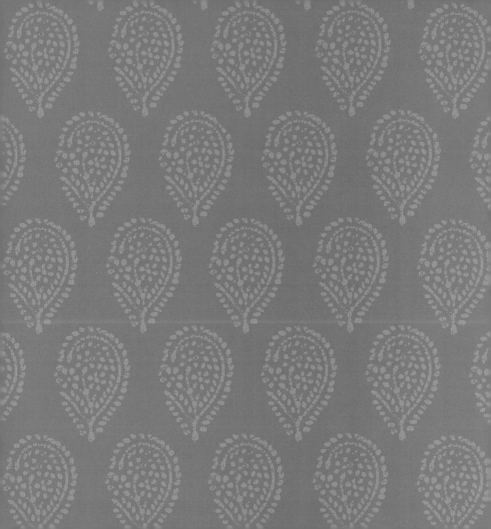

part II

kapha rhythms of winter and early spring

Winter and early spring, with dull skies and cold wet weather, comprise the heavy Kapha season, a time for consolidation and containment and a time to shelter from the cold in rest and reflection. Indeed, Kapha's qualities of nourishing and sustaining complement the season's inactivity, enabling the mind and body to quietly recharge in preparation for a new year ahead.

kapha

"The Kapha force is life-sustaining, lending qualities of strength and stamina to everything it inhabits."

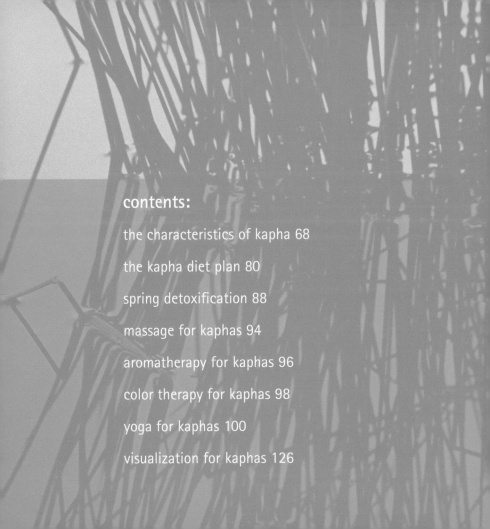

contents:

the characteristics of kapha

While Vata has the power to send the other doshas spinning out of balance, and Pitta, by presiding over the cell-nourishing digestive system, affects every part of the body, Kapha provides the substance and grounding everyone needs to be balanced. It lends its unique sustaining and cohesive qualities to everything we do. Kapha energy is composed of the elements water and earth. It has wet, cool, earthy, and oily qualities that bind, stabilize, lubricate, and sustain. The next five pages reveal how these qualities manifest themselves in the body, mind, and spirit of the Kapha individual.

the kapha body

Typically, Kapha types have a solid build. Kaphas often possess large, round faces and cute button noses. Hair is thick and lustrous, and skin is pale and perhaps oily. Kaphas have full mouths and large, round, attractive, even liquid, eyes. Teeth are generally strong and white, with healthy gums.

The seat of Kapha is in the chest, particularly in the lungs. Kapha energy is linked via its watery element to the body's lubrication and its secretions, and it also relates to the body's nourishment and supply systems.

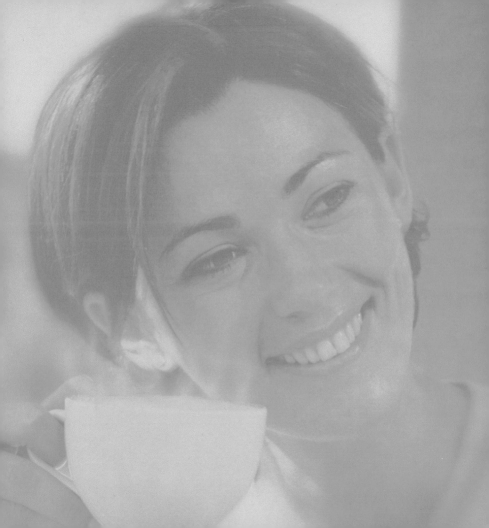

"Kapha has the greatest stamina of all the doshas."

From his or her earth element, the Kapha type inherits a solid reliability. Caring and compassionate, Kaphas can always be relied on in a crisis. They are often the people friends call when they require comfort, support, and tenderness or just need to talk out problems. Because Kapha individuals are centered, have a steady faith, and don't easily change their core beliefs, they find it easier than other dosha types to feel secure and content with life. Kaphas are very loyal and, being guided by a cohesive, sustaining force, have no trouble keeping their friends. The sustaining Kapha force also enhances longevity.

Kaphas are inherently patient, peaceful people. Full of empathy, they forgive more readily than Vatas and Pittas. They find it relatively easy to unburden themselves, and they don't hang on to baggage from the past.

the kapha season

Kapha reigns from the damp, cold days of very early winter through the early part of spring. Kapha times of day are from dawn to mid-morning and from early evening until about 10 p.m., and these are ideal times to counter Kapha's cold heaviness with some warming exercise to enliven a sluggish mind and body.

the kapha pace

There is a languidness about slow, graceful Kapha people. This still quality carries over to the sexual sphere: Kapha types may be slower to arouse but, once started, they enjoy great strength and stamina. Apart from being able to maintain friendships well, Kaphas consistently complete tasks at a steady pace. Kaphas may be slower than Pittas or Vatas to grasp new information, but they have a very reliable long–term memory.

kapha and stress

Under stress, Kaphas remain calm, unflappable, courageous, and protective of others. Tranquil, they are usually slower to react than other doshas, take time before responding, and are less likely than others to blurt out the wrong thing. Kapha people tend to be slow in making decisions, often preferring to preserve things just as they are, even if the status quo merits change.

kaphas and change

Kapha types are easygoing but don't like to be pushed too far beyond where they feel comfortable. They find it a challenge to get started and need to seek fresh physical and mental stimulation—unlike Vata, Kapha benefits from a change in routine. Kaphas' stable and sustaining qualities allow them to tolerate the fast-paced world much better than Pitta and Vata types. Ironically, if a Kapha can get moving and change where necessary, he or she has a good chance of surviving and thriving; it's just that Kaphas often are content to remain where they are.

the kapha sleep habit

Kapha is the dosha that governs sleep, so Kapha people sleep very well. Nothing disturbs them, but they risk sleeping too much and find it harder than other doshas to spring out of bed in the morning.

kaphas and weight

Kaphas put on weight easily. Unlike other dosha types, who are able to control weight by limiting food intake, Kaphas really need to combine dieting with exercise to get results. Kapha types don't have a strong hunger and are able to delay or miss meals without discomfort, but they tend to convert more calories to fat than

Pittas and Vatas do. On the bright side, Kapha has the greatest stamina of all the doshas—all of the stored energy means that once Kaphas get started, they don't tire easily.

the kapha time of life

Each dosha has an affinity with a particular time of life. The stage of life ruled by Kapha starts at conception, when the fetus is surrounded by amniotic fluid, and ends when the body reaches full development. The sustaining Kapha force gives babies and children their puppy fat and their ability to sleep easily and deeply.

symptoms of aggravated kapha

- greediness
- oversleeping
- lethargy
- heaviness
- avoidance of change

how to balance kapha

Kaphas need motivation and stimulation. Make variability, lightness, and change your mantras. While you like to stick to your routine, you should give it a gentle shake now and then to keep yourself from getting stuck in a rut. And once you do get moving, make sure to change direction again every so often. If you have a routine job, make sure you introduce action and variety into your free time. Above all, let excitement and challenge into your life! The following tips may help.

seek out the new
• Cultivate friendships with people from different walks of life.
• Be free-spirited, and get out and explore new activities, exhibitions, and parts of town.
• Stimulate the mind by attending lectures and investigating new ideas.
• Actively socialize with friends, and participate enthusiastically in shared activities.

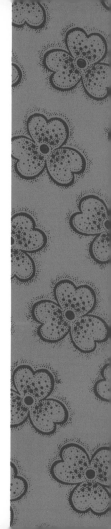

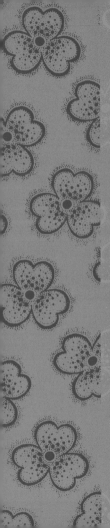

work out
- Get plenty of vigorous exercise.
- Take advantage of your great Kapha stamina and ability to exercise for longer periods than the other doshas, perhaps by opting for long power walks or jogs.
- Although your usual pace is slow and steady, extend yourself to explore your limits.
- Kaphas are good team players. Diplomatic and consistent, you do well in sports where you can let yourself be enthused by the energy of other players.
- Kapha types also enjoy active dance. If possible, partner up with a non-Kapha type and choose something faster than a slow waltz.

leap out of bed
- Sleep under light, warm covers, with the window open for fresh air.
- Don't sleep in. Set as many alarm clocks as you need to ensure that you wake up, and then practice bounding out of bed.
- Kapha rules the cool, stagnant, heavy morning time. Counter the Kapha influence with active, warming exercise at this time of day, and again at sunset.

- Unless you are ill or convalescing, never sleep during daylight hours. It will lower your energy for the rest of the day.
- Don't oversleep or overeat at any time.

relax actively
- The superfast modern world is Vata-increasing, and unflappable Kaphas have the ability to survive very well in it. Relaxation is important for everyone, but make sure that downtime is a break and not your whole lifestyle!

choose the right career
- Kaphas don't appreciate being hurried or pushed past their comfort zone—capitalize on the steady, stable, caring, and nurturing elements of your personality by selecting a job such as career counseling, nursing, construction, archeology, office management, administration, conservation, hospitality, or catering.

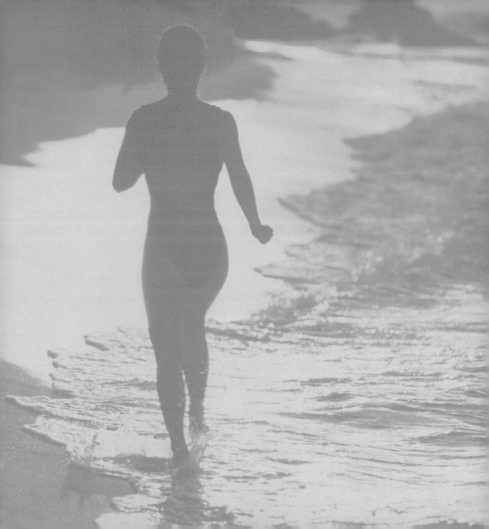

vacation vigorously

• Make vacations and weekends active, using them as opportunities to get moving.

• Select a warm climate and go walking or cycling.

• Restrict yourself to just a few lazy days of relaxation and spend the rest of the time visiting new places.

• Let each day bring fresh influences, new sights, and innovative activities.

live seasonally

• During winter, avoid sweet, sour, and salty foods. Favor light foods over heavy ones. Drink plenty of fresh ginger tea. Spring is a good time to detoxify *(see page 88)*.

• Be aware that spring is a vulnerable time for Kapha in the transition out of winter hibernation. Because of Kapha build up over winter, people are prone to catching colds, the flu, a fever, or hay fever in spring.

set goals

• Get to know yourself. Consider your special abilities and think about your purpose in life.

• Then write down your goals and decide on ways to move toward them.

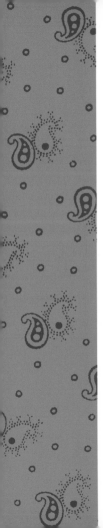

meditate daily
• To get the most out of the wonderful, consciousness-expanding practice of meditation, Kaphas should meditate when fully awake. Don't meditate in bed or while lying down or leaning against anything—you may be tempted to doze off.

• Kapha is strongly linked to the sense of smell, so you might enjoy using incense as part of your meditative ritual.

ways to throw kaphas off balance
• Overeating constantly
• Taking long snoozes after meals
• Sleeping during the day
• Indulging your tendency toward inertia
• Holding down a repetitive job, especially if it requires you to sit all day
• Watching hours of television at a stretch
• Taking drugs, especially sedatives
• Bottling up your feelings
• Eating lots of moist foods and sweet desserts

the kapha diet plan

To keep the Kapha dosha balanced and achieve ultimate well-being, adopt the following dos and don'ts of good eating.

kapha-balancing foods

Since Kapha has heavy, oily, and cold qualities, the best foods to balance excess Kapha are light, dry, and warm—specific types of foods that fulfill these criteria are detailed on the next four pages. Eat plenty of vegetables and lots of spices, and vary your choices. Feel free to skip breakfast or lunch if you wish. To avoid aggravating your dosha, keep away from all fried and greasy food, candy, and dairy products. And avoid overeating.

kapha-balancing tastes

Choose pungent, bitter, and astringent foods *(for rasa definitions, see pages 52–55)* whenever possible, and eat fewer sweet, sour, and salty foods.

dealing with vices

If you want to eat heavy, sticky food, do so before 6 p.m. The best time of the day to indulge is midday, and the best season is summer, when the active Pitta energy will assist your digestion.

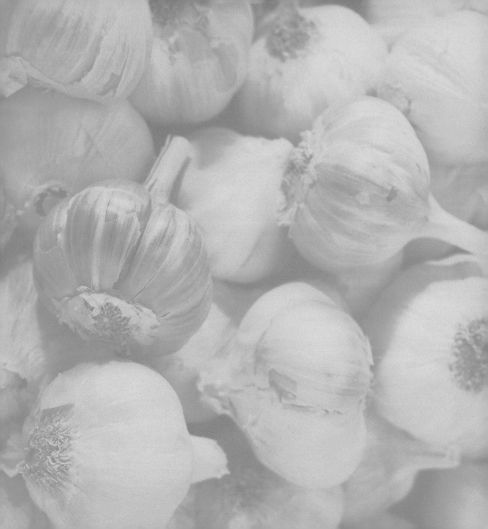

the kapha good food guide

grains
• Barley, buckwheat, corn, millet, and basmati and wild rice are good for Kaphas.

• Avoid wheat, quinoa, and white rice. Limit your pasta intake. Avoid bread—if you do eat it, have it toasted so it is less moist.

fruit and vegetables
• Dried or astringent fruit is good for Kapha types. Apples, apricots, cranberries, dried figs, mangoes, peaches, and pears are good.

• Avoid very juicy, sweet, or sour fruit.

• Kaphas can happily eat most vegetables, raw or cooked (but definitely not fried).

• Root vegetables, such as potatoes; pumpkin; and very juicy vegetables, like squash or tomatoes, are slightly less beneficial than other vegetables.

meat and animal products
• Kaphas don't require a lot of meat. If you do eat meat, make sure it's cooked in a dry way (roasted or baked) and not fried. Kaphas do well to reduce consumption of red meat. Better animal products for Kapha are chicken, eggs, seafood, and venison.

legumes

• Legumes provide a good source of protein, but Kaphas need less protein than other doshas.

• Black lentils, kidney beans, soy beans, and tofu are rather heavy for Kaphas. Instead, choose black beans, miso, mung beans, pinto beans, red lentils, and tempeh.

nuts and seeds

• In general, nuts weigh heavily on Kapha—avoid them.
• Eat sunflower and pumpkin seeds just occasionally.

dairy

• Don't eat a lot of dairy: It has heavy, oily, and cooling qualities that can aggravate Kapha.
• Goat's milk is better than cow's milk, and cottage cheese is better than other cheeses. If you must drink milk, add fresh ginger to lighten it.

oils

• Keep consumption of any oils to a minimum; Kapha is oily enough without adding more.
• Use almond, corn, or sunflower oil in small amounts.

spices and condiments
- All spices, especially garlic and ginger, are great for Kapha types.
- Salt is a seasoning to limit.
- Avoid lime pickles, mayonnaise, and vinegar.

sweeteners
- Avoid sweeteners as much as possible.
- When sweetening is necessary, use natural honey or fruit juice concentrates, which can pacify Kapha.

alcohol
- Wine is better than beer or spirits; apple cider is tolerated.

drinks
- Occasional cups of coffee or black tea can be beneficial to Kapha types. Hot, spiced soy drinks and grain coffees are suitable alternatives.
- Choose apricot, carrot, sweet cherry, cranberry, grape, mango, and mixed vegetable juices. Avoid grapefruit, orange, papaya, and pineapple juice.
- Herbal teas, such as those made with chamomile, chicory, dandelion, fenugreek, ginger, lemongrass, sage, and yarrow, are good.
- Avoid carbonated drinks, iced teas, and very cold drinks.

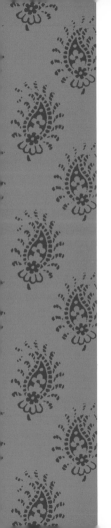

kapha menu ideas

These are not complete recipes, but rather are quick ideas for ways to combine ingredients to make the most of the Kapha dosha. Good times of the day and year to eat them are also suggested.

seasonal eating
During the Kapha season of winter and early spring, eat plenty of buckwheat and millet; garbanzo beans, kidney beans, mung beans, and red lentils; and carrots, green vegetables, mushrooms, onions, peas, red beets, spinach, and turnips.

ideas for breakfast
• Puffed millet, oats, rice, and wheat
• Rolled barley-based muesli
Accompany all the above with goat's milk or soya milk spiced with cardamom
• Fresh fruit during the warm seasons
• Oat bran muffins
• Poached eggs.

ideas for lunch
- Cornbread
- Rice crackers
- Rye crackers
- Sandwich on rye bread with carrot, beet, lettuce, and tomato
- Salad of light leafy greens, such as lettuce, arugula, spinach, and bitter greens like chicory, endive, and radicchio.

ideas for dinner
- Rice and light vegetable stir fry—use minimal oil and Kapha-pacifying vegetables, such as broccoli, cauliflower, and eggplant
- Basmati rice with vegetables and tempeh
- Millet with steamed vegetables
- Vegetable curries with beans, such as black beans, mung beans, pinto beans, adzuki beans, black-eyed peas, garbanzo beans, or red lentils
- Large green salad; for interest, add a sliced pear or some dried apricots and a sprinkling of sunflower seeds
- Raw vegetable salad with sprouts or olives; don't eat it cold from the refrigerator but let the ingredients warm up to room temperature first

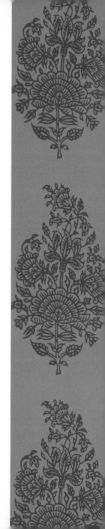

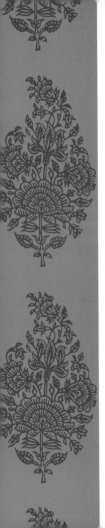

- Occasional bean nachos with chili and very little dairy
- Occasional portions of falafel in pita bread with salad.

ideas for dessert
- Fruit in season
- Fruit salad
- Fruit cobbler (in winter)
- Stewed apricots, figs, pears, or prunes (in winter)
- Baked apples (in winter).

ideas for snacks
- Popcorn (popped without oil or butter)
- Olives
- Miso soup.

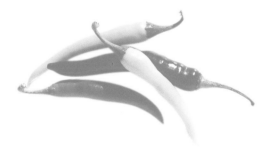

spring detoxification

Spring, when all living things emerge from winter hibernation, is a good time for detoxification. After the Kapha winter, many Hindus traditionally fast, often by eating only fruit or non-salty foods for up to 9 days. The Kapha constitution responds well to a detox diet of freshly steamed vegetables at this time; a khichadi diet *(see pages 218–19)* is another good way to detoxify body and mind, with the help of the triphala herbal mix *(see page 153)*.

If you stay in harmony by eating and living according to the seasons and your constitution, you will experience a minimum of spring-time aggravation. However, if dietary excess and the Kapha winter have contributed to a buildup of ama (toxins), weight gain, hay fever, or respiratory congestion, you may want to purify your system with a full ayurvedic detoxification, known as panchakarma *(see overleaf)*.

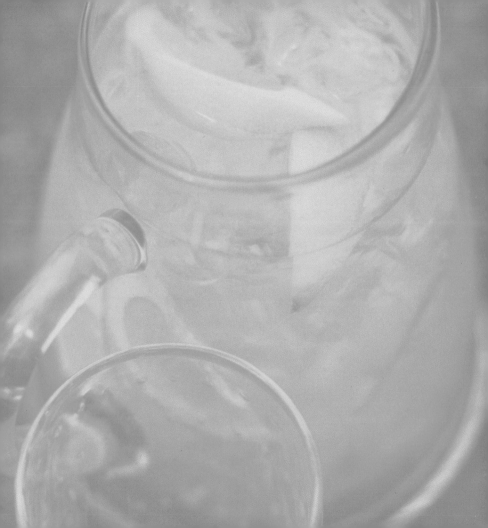

panchakarma

The ayurvedic deep-cleansing process called *panchakarma* releases toxins from the cells, purifies the body, and balances the doshas for better health. Alongside physical purification, panchakarma seeks to transform consciousness, and some emotional release can result from this detoxification process. While panchakarma should not be traumatic, it may be emotionally challenging, and you can experience deep tiredness as the body begins to heal. Keeping to a good diet appropriate to your dosha and getting plenty of rest are essential while the panchakarma therapies work deeply to nourish the body and encourage it to release toxins. Apart from helping in the healing of previously entrenched diseases, panchakarma may offer long-lasting emotional benefits, such as improvements in how you view life and interact with those around you.

A panchakarma treatment given by an ayurvedic doctor includes a special diet, such as khichadi *(see pages 218–219)*; daily medicated oil massage; and other therapies—including herbal steaming, application of natural drawing agents to the skin, or a warm flow massage to the forehead using oil or buttermilk. Other possible treatments include forms of therapeutic purgation, elimination, or enemas, each to rebalance the appropriate dosha.

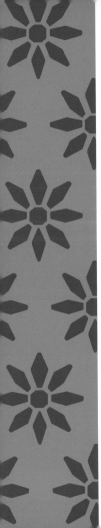

Because it is such a deep process, a full panchakarma treatment is not suitable for everyone and must be performed only under the supervision of an ayurvedic doctor experienced in panchakarma. However, you can safely adapt certain elements of the panchakarma for a home-style detoxification that rests the digestive system and cleanses the body. Try the following gentle program.

do-it-yourself panchakarma

• Take a week off from work, or close your doors to the world for a long weekend.

• Get plenty of rest and take each activity and treatment slowly. Minimize sensory distractions, such as television or music.

• Follow a khichadi diet *(see pages 218–19)* for 3 to 7 days. Keep the body well hydrated with spring water and herbal teas, and cut out coffee, black tea, and other stimulants.

• Give yourself a daily oil massage, following the instructions appropriate to your dosha.

• Take long, contemplative strolls outdoors, but stay out of the sun and wind.

• Practice gentle yoga asanas appropriate to your dosha, and meditate.

managing your weight

More than Pittas and Vatas, Kaphas must take care to avoid putting on weight. Obesity is linked to an increased risk of many chronic ailments—such as heart disease, cancers, diabetes, hypertension, and arthritis—so try to maintain your weight within the average range for your height. Diet is a particularly important way to tackle weight gain for Kaphas. Follow the ayurvedic eating guidelines on pages 56-59, and make sure you eat according to your constitution. These thoughts may also help.

think before you eat

• Examine your relationship with food and the emotions you experience when you eat. Do you eat from boredom, for comforting emotional sustenance, or with anger, despair, or defiance? See a counselor if you feel that emotional baggage lies at the root of a self-destructive relationship with food.

• Eat two meals daily and never snack. The Kapha digestive system efficiently and slowly extracts maximum nutrients from your food, so don't put in another load until the stomach has emptied—this takes about four hours. If you still feel hungry after a meal, wait 20 minutes before taking a second helping.

• Rather than using food for emotional comfort, think of positive, nonharmful replacements, such as the company of friends, or outdoor activities.

• It's better to eat to live than to live to eat. If you constantly think about what, when, or where you'll next eat, focus on being more active. When eating, concentrate on savoring each mouthful.

• While nourishment from food is important, check that you're not trying to energize with calories when you are really lacking mental inspiration.

• Eat according to your ayurvedic constitution. Avoid sweet, sour, and salty foods; fried and greasy food; desserts; and dairy products. Eat plenty of vegetables and lots of spices, and don't get stuck in a rut—vary the selection. Pungent, bitter, and astringent foods *(see pages 52-55)* are best for Kapha.

• Dine according to the seasons. In winter, balance the Kapha force with warming, light foods. Don't succumb to the temptation of heavy, moist foods when the season is already heavy and moist.

massage for kaphas

Firm massage stimulates the function of the organs, reduces fluid retention, and encourages the breakdown of fat cells to detoxify the body. Kapha types benefit from a weekly self-massage using a dry powder, such as talcum powder, or a light, cold-pressed oil like corn, mustard, safflower, or sweet almond. (Apricot kernel, jojoba, and wheatgerm oils are suitable for all dosha types.) You can follow the instructions for oil massage on page 222—as a Kapha, you'll benefit from the Easy Abdominal Massage on page 223, and Indian Head Massage on pages 154–55, as well as from the stimulating massage outlined on these pages.

energy-balancing massage

This brief, invigorating massage is suitable for all constitutional types and stimulates the energy meridians of the body. It's particularly good for Kaphas, as it is invigorating and no oil is necessary. You can remain fully clothed; just take off your shoes.

❶ Sit comfortably on the floor. Place the sole of one foot face up on the thigh of the other leg. Make loose fists with your hands and, with floppy wrists, pound the sole of the foot. When you feel a nice tingling sensation, switch legs and work on the other foot.

❷ Bend your legs up in front of you. Using a medium pressure, pound up the muscles on the inner calf, and then those on the inner thigh. Repeat three times. Then pound briskly up the outer calf and outer thigh. Repeat three times. Work on the other leg.

❸ Rest the back of one hand on your leg and pound the palm with the other hand. Then pound three times up the inner arm from wrist to armpit. Finally, pound three times up the outer arm from wrist to shoulder. Change sides to work on the other arm.

❹ Briskly pound the muscles on the tops of both shoulders, using a pressure that feels good to you.

❺ Pitter-patter your fingers over your face and scalp.

❻ Tarzan-like, pummel your chest with two loose fists.

❼ Kneel up, lean forward, and pummel your buttocks and thighs. Sit back down.

❽ Now, sit comfortably with eyes closed, and observe how alive your body feels.

aromatherapy for kaphas

Essential oils that are warming and stimulating help balance Kapha. Select those with an aroma that appeals to you, and don't stick with the same mix: Vary your choice to reflect the day and season and your time of life. To use essential oils, add a few drops to your bath, oil burner, pillow pad, or massage oil.

Cautions: Don't take essential oils internally or apply them undiluted to the skin. Do not use essential oils while pregnant or breastfeeding: For massage during these times, use the carrier oil alone.

making massage oils

When using essential oils in a blend for massage, use a Kapha-pacifying carrier oil, such as corn, mustard, safflower, or sweet almond. Add 10 drops total of essential oils (either one oil or a blend of two or more) to 20 ml carrier oil.

aromatherapy oils to uplift kapha

• basil • bergamot • camphor • cinnamon • eucalyptus • juniper • lemon • orange • peppermint • rosemary • sage

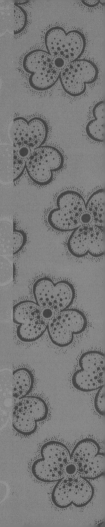

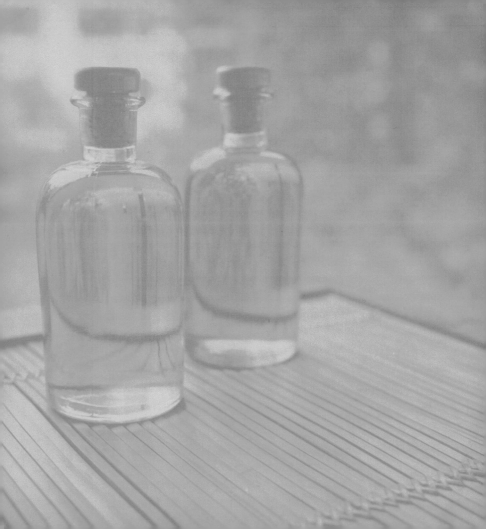

color therapy for kaphas

Each color has physiological and psychological effects caused by the vibrations it emits. Read about which colors help rebalance Kapha, and then select a fitting color and surround yourself with it—wear it, visualize it, eat, breathe, and drink it!

good kapha colors

• Warm red is a great color for Kapha as it stimulates and brings energy and vitality to this slower-moving dosha.

• Turquoise gets Kapha involved and moving should the Kapha force cause stagnation.

• Magenta is another useful color: It helps you let go of old patterns and initiate new ways of being when change is needed.

• Orange is a stimulating color that embodies a dancing energy, enhancing lightness, movement, and release. Warm orange, because it lies between red and yellow, wards off mental sluggishness and brings joy while you work.

• Green relates to Kapha's water element, while blue echoes its earth element. As an all-around balancer, green harmonizes any system and is particularly valued in the treatment of Kapha-dominant conditions, such as growths and tumors.

color solutions

Now that you know which color to select for which purpose, use these ideas to introduce color into every part of your life.

• To energize water with a beneficial color, wrap colored cellophane around a glass pitcher filled with water. Place it in the sun for a few hours, and then sip solarized water that has imbibed the vibrations of your color.

• Breathe your color: Visualize drawing in the chosen color as you inhale, then exhale its complementary color *(see pages 190–91)*.

• Wear the color in your clothing. If you don't feel daring, simply add a scarf of the appropriate color to one of your regular outfits. Wear jewelry containing gemstones in the color you adopt.

• Paint your chosen color onto your walls, or incorporate it into furnishings in every room—try throws, drapes, bed linens, cushions, and tablecloths.

• Colorize a room by replacing clear light bulbs with colored ones, or by placing colored cellophane over window panes.

yoga for kaphas

To counter their natural lethargy, Kapha types need stimulating, heat-building exercise that requires plenty of effort. If it makes you sweat, great! Bring movement to your yoga practice by flowing in and out of the postures, taking only short rests between each asana. Don't lose momentum with long recovery breaks. Although you won't enjoy being pushed beyond your limit, you're not put off by a new exercise regimen if it is built up over time in a slow, steady way, so aim for this approach to yoga practice. Since Kaphas tend to have shorter bones and bulkier bodies than the other doshas, you may feel initially that you lack the grace you would like; with practice, watch how this, too, improves.

Each yoga pose is beneficial for the bodymind, but the poses on pages 102–23 are especially good for Kaphas. *(For Vata, see pages 226–45; for Pitta, see pages 160–81).* Also try out the yoga poses recommended for the other doshas. These poses can be valuable for Kaphas, particularly if they are practiced in the invigorating, Kapha-balancing manner suggested.

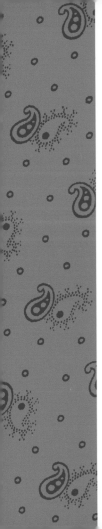

yoga breathing

Yoga breathing exercises are outlined for each dosha. While the exercises may feel subtler than other forms of regular exercise, as if they might have less obvious effects, they contribute to health in a profound way. Your breath, vital force, and energy levels are intrinsically connected. (In fact, yogis have the same word for both—*prana*.) Deep, conscious breathing that fully expands the lungs is a powerful energizing tool.

On another level, yogis have observed that the breath is a mirror of the mind. Any alteration in one will affect the other. Good breathing is reassuring, soothing, and healing. Exercises that cool, warm, energize, or calm the system are given for each dosha *(for Kapha, see pages 124–25, for Pitta, see pages 182–87, and for Vata, see pages 246–49)*. In addition, everyone can benefit from Nadi Sodhana (pages 183–84). Breathing exercises, like yoga postures, are best practiced on an empty stomach. Lie down to rest in Savasana (pages 244–45) afterward. Take things easy, especially in the beginning, and remember that the breath should never feel unnaturally forced.

surya namaskar (SUN SALUTATION)

Surya namaskar is a dynamic series of postures that is a
wonderful way to start a practice. Its folding and unfolding
movements are performed with one breath per action, and
the flowing form gives a Kapha an energizing kick start.

❶ Stand tall with feet
together, and place
your palms together
in front of the chest
in Namaste prayer
position.

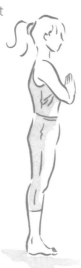

❷ Inhale, and stretch
the arms
overhead.

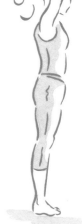

3 Exhale, and fold forward to bring the hands to the floor next to the feet, in Uttanasana *(see pages 108–9).*

4 Inhale, tilt the pelvis forward, flatten the back, and look along the floor in front of you.

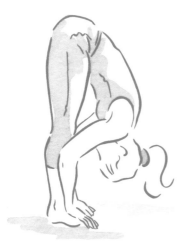

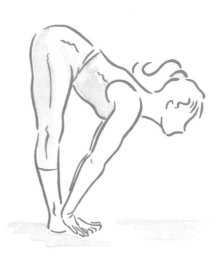

surya namaskar (SUN SALUTATION)

⑤ Exhale, and step your feet one by one or jump both feet back together. Bring your body into one straight line from shoulders to heels.

⑥ Still on the same exhalation, bend the elbows and drop the chest, chin, and knees to the ground.

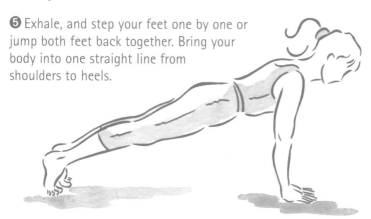

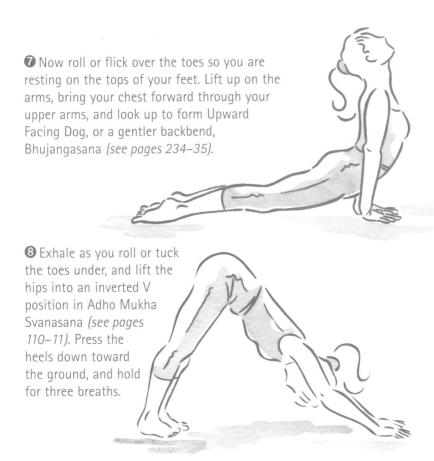

7 Now roll or flick over the toes so you are resting on the tops of your feet. Lift up on the arms, bring your chest forward through your upper arms, and look up to form Upward Facing Dog, or a gentler backbend, Bhujangasana *(see pages 234–35)*.

8 Exhale as you roll or tuck the toes under, and lift the hips into an inverted V position in Adho Mukha Svanasana *(see pages 110–11)*. Press the heels down toward the ground, and hold for three breaths.

surya namaskar (SUN SALUTATION)

❾ On an inhalation, step or jump the feet forward. With fingertips or palms to the floor, lift your chest away from your thighs and look forward.

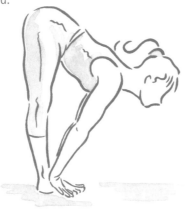

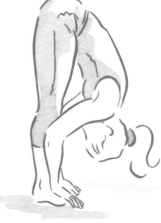

❿ Exhale and fold forward to Uttanasana. Use your arms to help lever you down into a deep forward bend, as in step 3.

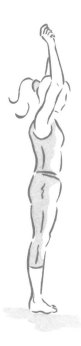

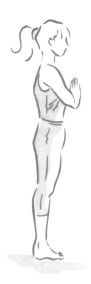

11 Inhale, and stand up with arms stretched overhead, as in step 2.

12 Exhale, and lower the arms. Repeat all 12 steps of the sun salutation, building up to eight rounds.

uttanasana (STANDING FORWARD BEND)

Standing poses involve large muscle groups from the entire body and are useful not only to Kaphas, but to any dosha type. Forward bending helps Kapha tone and stimulate the digestive system.

❶ Stand with feet hip-width apart and hands on hips. Extend your torso up so the top of the breastbone moves away from the pubic bone.

❷ Keeping the knees bent, crease in at the top of the thighs to fold the torso over the legs. Keep the chest open by not rounding the back. Depending on your flexibility, grasp your shins or ankles, or loop your fingers and thumb around the big toes.

❸ Remain in the pose, using each exhalation to work toward straightening your legs. Return upright on an exhalation. To make the pose more challenging, start with the feet together. Then, by activating the front thigh muscles, bring your weight forward so the hip joints are aligned directly over the ankle joints.

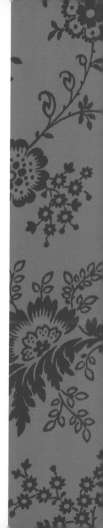

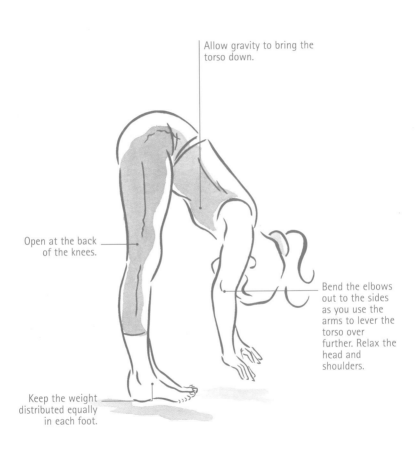

Allow gravity to bring the torso down.

Open at the back of the knees.

Bend the elbows out to the sides as you use the arms to lever the torso over further. Relax the head and shoulders.

Keep the weight distributed equally in each foot.

adho mukha svanasana

(DOWNWARD FACING DOG)

An excellent full-body stretch, this asana warms the whole body while building strength and flexibility. Kaphas should practice this posture between standing poses, such as the Triangle poses Trikonasana *(see pages 166–67)* and Parivrtta Trikonasana *(see pages 168–69)*.

❶ Begin on all fours. Place the hands on the floor about 8 in. (20 cm) in front of the shoulders. The middle fingers should be facing straight ahead. Check that your feet and knees are as wide apart as your hipbones.

❷ Tuck your toes under and lift your hips high. Move your hips up and back, away from the wrists, so that pressure moves away from the palms. Stretch your heels down toward the floor to straighten both legs fully.

❸ Hold for five to ten steady breaths. Then bend the knees down to the floor, press the buttocks back toward the heels, and rest with your forehead on the floor.

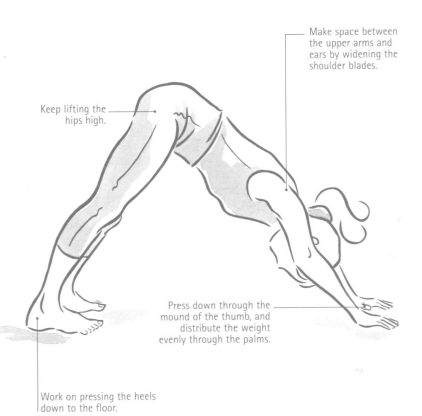

Make space between the upper arms and ears by widening the shoulder blades.

Keep lifting the hips high.

Press down through the mound of the thumb, and distribute the weight evenly through the palms.

Work on pressing the heels down to the floor.

setu bandha sarvangasana

(BRIDGE POSE—HALF BACKARCH)

This warming and energizing pose helps regulate the function of the thyroid gland; in doing so, it works to balance the basal metabolic rate, which is especially beneficial for Kaphas. After this pose, Kaphas should practice Bhujangasana (pages 234–35) and Dhanurasana (pages 172–73), which also help ease problems such as sinus or lung congestion, asthma, and headaches. Stretch the spine in Adho Mukha Svanasana (pages 110–11).

❶ Lie on your back with knees bent up. Place your heels about 6 in. (15 cm) from your buttocks, feet parallel and placed as wide apart as your hipbones.

❷ Slowly lift your hips while lengthening through the lower back. Then tuck the shoulders under one by one and bring the breastbone closer to the chin.

❸ Hold the pose for up to ten breaths. To come down, slowly roll down in sections from the top of the spine. Rest, and repeat twice more.

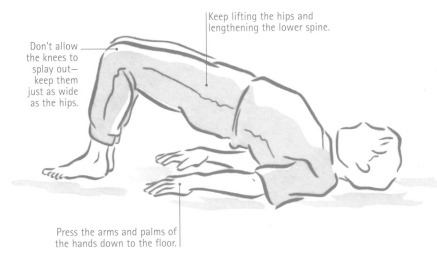

Keep lifting the hips and lengthening the lower spine.

Don't allow the knees to splay out— keep them just as wide as the hips.

Press the arms and palms of the hands down to the floor.

sarvangasana

(SHOULDER STAND)

This pose brings a nourishing supply of blood to the thyroid gland, which is valuable for Kaphas. Follow shoulder stands with a twist, such as Bharadvajasana (pages 118–19).

Cautions: Do not practice this pose if you have a heart condition, high blood pressure, or eye or ear problems. If you have had previous neck injuries or are pregnant, seek advice from an experienced yoga teacher first.

❶ Fold a blanket into a 2 ft. x 3 ft. (60 cm x 90 cm) rectangle. Lie with your head and upper back on the cushioned surface. Use your abdominal muscles to bring your legs up and overhead. You should be slightly folded forward from the hips, with the arms taking a fair amount of pressure. Begin with 25 breaths in this pose and, over time, build your holding time to several minutes.

❷ To come out of the pose, roll the spine down to the floor in stages, then use the abdominal muscles to lower the legs. Lie flat and rest for a short time.

FOLLOW WITH:

janu shirshasana
SEATED HEAD-TO-KNEE, PAGES
238–39
pashchimottanasana
SEATED FORWARD BEND, PAGES
174–75,
yogamudrasana, SEALING POSE,
PAGES 242–43, AND
upavistha konasana, OPEN ANGLE,
PAGES 176–77.

Check that the neck feels relatively soft and relaxed—it should not be strained tight.

Make sure there is no tension in the face.

Support the body weight equally through both arms.

halasana (PLOW POSE)

Practice this asana after completing step 2 of
Sarvangasana *(pages 114–15)*. It shares similar effects with
the shoulder stand and should be followed by the same
complementary poses.

Cautions: Do not practice this pose if you have a heart
condition, high blood pressure, or eye or ear problems. If
you have had previous neck injuries or are pregnant, seek
advice from an experienced yoga teacher first.

❶ From the Shoulder Stand *(see pages 114–15)*, lower your
legs toward the ground behind your head. Don't over-
stretch the neck, but support your back with your hands.

❷ To deepen the pose, roll more onto the tips of the
shoulders, interlace your fingers, and stretch your arms.
Start with ten breaths and build up to a few minutes.

❸ Come out of the pose with control. Roll your spine down
to the floor in stages. With your back on the floor, use your
abdominal muscles to lower both legs and lie flat.

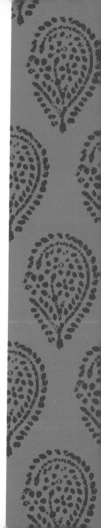

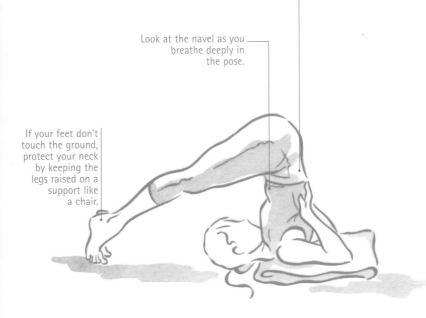

Work on lengthening the torso in a straight line from neck to tailbone.

Look at the navel as you breathe deeply in the pose.

If your feet don't touch the ground, protect your neck by keeping the legs raised on a support like a chair.

bharadvajasana on a chair

(SAGE TWIST ON A CHAIR)

Kaphas tend to have a lack of abdominal tone. Twists
help tone the abdomen while feeding the digestive fire,
detoxifying the system, and boosting a sluggish
metabolism.

❶ Sit on the side of a chair with your right hip toward the
back of it. Place your knees and feet about hip-width apart.

❷ To help elongate the torso, raise your arms straight up
in the air. Without slumping, keep this lift as you lower
your arms, twist around to the right, and hold the chair.

❸ Work on twisting from the bottom up. Start at the
pelvis by drawing the lower abdominal muscles around to
the right, then bring the upper abdominal muscles into
the twist. Next, move the whole ribcage around, then the
shoulders, neck, and eyes. This right-sided twist
stimulates the ascending colon. After holding for ten
breaths, release, and change to a left-sided twist to
stimulate the descending colon.

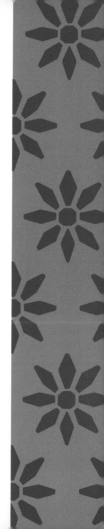

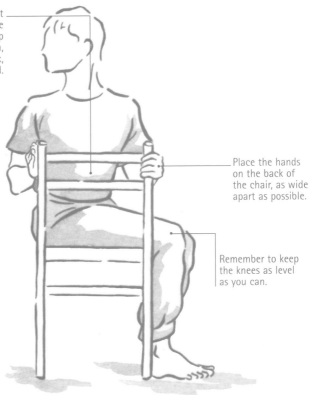

Intensify the twist starting from the base of the spine. Work up through the abdomen, ribcage, shoulders, neck, and head.

Place the hands on the back of the chair, as wide apart as possible.

Remember to keep the knees as level as you can.

urdhva prasarita padasana

(UPWARD EXTENDED FOOT POSE)

This abdominal strengthener tones the abdomen and nourishes the digestive fire; both actions are valuable for Kapha constitutions. If you find working with straight legs too challenging, or if you experience back pain, bend the knees during the pose. If you prefer more challenge, stretch your arms overhead along the floor as you practice.

❶ Lie on your back with arms by your side, palms down. As you inhale, lift the right leg in the air. On an exhalation, slowly lower the leg. Raise the left leg on an inhalation, and exhale it down. Repeat six times.

❷ On an inhalation, raise both legs together so that they are at a 90 degree angle to your torso. As you exhale, lower them by 30 degrees. Hold for five breaths. Exhale and lower them another 30 degrees; hold the position again for five breaths. Lower the legs until they are just above the floor; hold for five breaths, and then release the legs down. Repeat this double leg lift three more times.

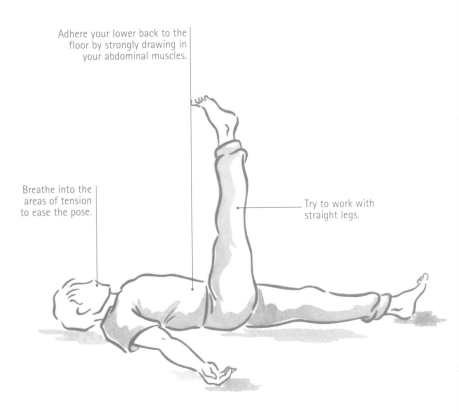

Adhere your lower back to the floor by strongly drawing in your abdominal muscles.

Breathe into the areas of tension to ease the pose.

Try to work with straight legs.

navasana (BOAT POSE)

Kaphas can develop determination by strengthening the willpower center at the abdomen with this toning pose. The asana also improves digestion, encourages toxins to disperse, and assists the workings of the pancreas. Always finish your yoga session with Savasana *(see pages 110-11)*. Try to stay alert and attuned to the progressive relaxation of your body.

❶ Sit with both legs in front of you. Lean back on your hands and lift the legs, with knees bent and shins parallel to the floor. To keep the chest from sinking, lift it a little.

❷ Stretch the arms forward, parallel to your shins, and gaze at your toes. Hold for five breaths, before resting and repeating three times.

❸ For the more challenging full Boat Pose, straighten both legs in the air. Gaze at your pointed toes. To increase the degree of difficulty, move the legs away from your lifted chest. Hold for five breaths, and repeat three times.

Look at the toes, keeping the face relaxed.

Keep the arms outstretched and parallel to the floor.

Don't round the back; instead take the small of the back in toward the navel and up.

breathing for kaphas

Yoga breathing features some abdominal stimulating exercises that suit Kapha types perfectly. Kaphas also benefit from warming Ujjayi (pages 246–47), balancing Nadi Sodhana (pages 183–84), and calming Bhramari (page 248).

Cautions: Practice Kapalabhati and Uddiyana on an empty stomach. Don't practice these techniques if you suffer from ulceration, hernia, heart problems, vertigo, or high blood pressure. Never practice these during pregnancy or menstruation. If you experience dizziness or faintness, ask an experienced yoga teacher to check your practice.

kapalabhati (CLEANSING BREATH)
This technique uses a quick, forced exhalation that is incredibly revitalizing. As it stimulates the abdominal region, it is good for anyone who needs to improve muscle tone.

❶ Sit comfortably erect, either cross-legged or on your heels. Place your hands on your knees. Breathe normally. Exhale forcibly and quickly through the nose, then relax the abdominal muscles and let the inhalation come in

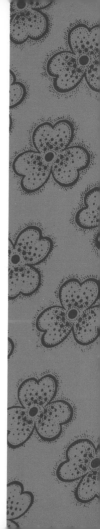

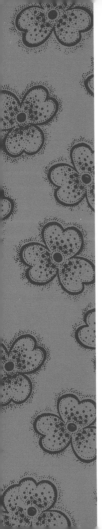

naturally, without force, through the nose. Repeat 10-20 breaths like this, at the rate of one breath per second.

❷ Return to quiet, steady breathing, and take as many breaths as you need to return to normal. When you feel ready, begin the second round of Kapalabhati. Rest, taking regular breaths, before repeating one final round.

uddiyana (ABDOMINAL GRIP)
Uddiyana is good for people of all doshas. It provides a stimulating workout for the organs by stretching and momentarily compressing them.

❶ From a standing position, exhale fully to empty the lungs as much as possible. Do not forcibly push the air out, just let it flow out in a leisurely, relaxed manner. As you come to the end of the exhalation, bend forward a little, and place your hands on your bent knees.

❷ Press the chin toward the throat. With the lungs empty, pull up the diaphragm muscle strongly. Finally, release the chin from the throat, stand up, and inhale.

visualization for kaphas

This visualization is just the thing to get a lethargic Kapha moving, and it uplifts people of all doshas when they are feeling sluggish. Of the many effective visualization techniques, Trataka *(see pages 252-53)*, Meditation *(see pages 250-51)*, Sanctuary Visualization *(see pages 188-89)*, and Color Breathing *(see pages 190-91)* are most beneficial for Kaphas.

energizing visualization

❶ Lie flat on your back, or get into Breathing Easy Position *(see Savasana II, pages 180-1)*. Each time you inhale through the nose, visualize yourself breathing in pure, vibrant energy.

❷ From the nose, let this positive revitalizing force travel down to the solar plexus, just above your navel. With each inhalation, feel this special energy concentrating around the solar plexus, forming a dense core.

❸ As you continue breathing steadily, feel the energy begin to spiral around, filling up the abdomen. Let each

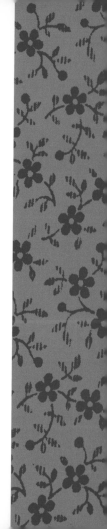

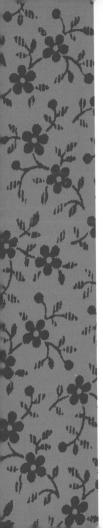

inhalation feed this swirl of energy, and feel it beginning to fill your entire torso. You are filling with vitality and strength; your body is becoming wonderfully energized.

❹ As you continue slow, deep breathing, let this verve spill over into your limbs, and feel them becoming stronger and lighter.

❺ As the energy consolidates in the body, let it filter into and fill the head. Your nervous system and brain are uplifted and infused with stamina.

❻ Stay with this breathing until you are completely energized. Filled with this vibrant force, let yourself become enthusiastic about life and your ability to tackle every task joyfully. Feel that you have plenty of energy to carry you through the day.

❼ When it's time to come out of the exercise, visualize sealing your special energy within. Then take your arms overhead along the floor and enjoy a slow stretch out from toes to fingertips.

part III

pitta rhythms of late spring and summer

Pitta, hot and explosive, starts to build during the spring as the weather warms up. The fire element of Pitta, like springtime, has transformative qualities—visualize a naked branch breaking out into leaves and blossom, or the miraculous development of a seed into a plant. Like a forest fire, Pitta is most likely to cause problems in the middle of summer when temperatures reach their maximum. Late summer is a time to rest in the shade and enjoy nature's abundance.

pitta

"Pitta types have discriminating, sharp minds and a bold confidence that makes them great leaders."

contents:

the characteristics of pitta

Pitta is composed of the elements fire and water. Like fire, Pitta is penetrating, piercing, quick, and strong. Fire, like Pitta, radiates heat, and when it meets water, steam is created. Pitta types, therefore, get overheated more quickly than the other doshas and prefer cool climates—these are the people who leave windows open and roll up their sleeves even in winter.

the pitta body

Pittas have well-proportioned bodies, and their weight doesn't usually fluctuate by more than a few pounds. Their facial features are average in size with few irregularities, although you might notice a rather penetrating gaze. Pitta coloring, when compared with that of other members of the family, is relatively fair. Hair is often fine, soft, and straight; baldness, early graying, and thinning also signal a Pitta influence. Freckly redheads and florid-skinned people are often Pitta types. Other signs of Pitta include numerous moles and skin that burns easily in the sun.

TO READ ABOUT **kapha**, SEE PAGES 65-127;
AND **vata,** SEE PAGES 193-253.

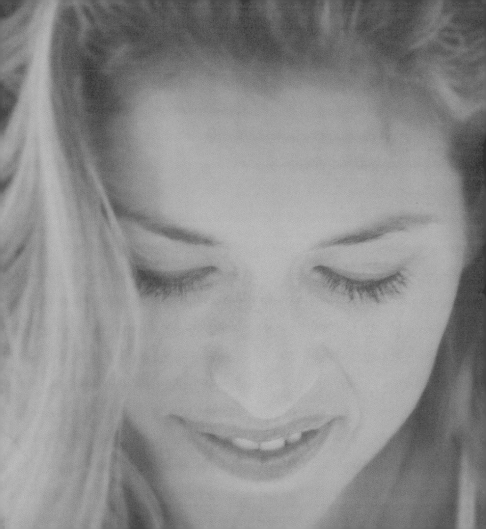

the pitta attitude

Confident, determined, and cheerful, Pitta types have sharp, discriminating minds and the ability to focus thoughts and energies very effectively. Precise and orderly Pittas exhibit a keen intellect and enthusiasm for learning, and they grasp new information easily. They are enterprising types, good at manipulating information to their advantage. They make great public speakers, as they are accomplished at thinking on their feet and quick to respond. Fortunately, their responses are usually accurate, too. Guided by a grand plan, Pitta people don't fritter money away on little things, and they happily spend it on luxuries. Pittas are sensitive to heat and light, so you will often spot them in designer sunglasses.

the pitta pace

Brave, ambitious, and passionate about what they do, Pitta people carry themselves well and move with a determined stride. As courageous visionaries, they may be demanding, critical, or stubborn. They are intense too, prone to being argumentative and to imposing their will on others. Such bold confidence makes Pittas great leaders. Pitta passion carries into the sexual arena, where Pitta types have a strong sex drive and, in bed and out, a healthy stamina.

pitta and stress

While Vatas react to stress by becoming anxious and fearful, and Kaphas dig their heels in, Pittas tend to become angry and impatient. However, because of Pitta's self-control, these emotions aren't always visible. Although hot-headed, Pittas keep the larger goal in mind and so are not at the mercy of changeable moods like Vata people are.

the pitta mind and memory

Pitta types have excellent powers of concentration. They easily recall information which furthers their aims, but unfortunately sometimes the birthdays of their nearest and dearest can be forgotten. Pitta-dominant types also have a powerful reasoning capacity and a strong intellect.

the pitta appetite

Because the seat of Pitta is the small intestine, the digestive system is where the force of a Pitta person's will arises. Pittas have a strong appetite and can't tolerate missing meals. The Pitta dosha deals with all metabolic processes. It provides the heat of fire to digest food and transform its nutrients into energy. Pitta is integral to the creation of thirst and hunger, and to the maintenance of body temperature.

the pitta season
Starting when the weather heats up in late spring, the Pitta season runs through the summer. Transformative Pitta energy guides nature's regeneration during spring, when plants bud and flower and fruits are growing. Pitta is most active at the hottest time of the day—midday. Pitta also rules the hours on either side of midnight, and the best time for Pittas to fall asleep at night is before 10 p.m., the hour at which Pitta takes over from Kapha.

the pitta time of life
Each dosha has an affinity with a particular time of life. The stage of life ruled by Pitta runs from adulthood through to late middle age. This is the most productive part of life, a time of active achievement in the workplace and at home.

symptoms of aggravated pitta
- irritation
- mood swings
- anger
- frustration
- jealousy
- criticism
- argumentativeness

"Pitta is most active at the hottest time of the day—midday."

how to balance pitta

Because Pitta contains the element fire, you need to keep cool. During the Pitta summer season, wear cool, natural-fiber clothing and stay out of the sun. Cool your temper, too, by balancing your competitiveness, keeping an eye on your controlling nature, and taking time out to relax; some of the following tips will help. Pittas are gifted with strong digestion, but if you abuse it, it will suffer with age, so eat regularly and eat foods appropriate to your dosha.

eat regular meals

- Eat regularly to avoid dizziness, nausea, or irritability. Three meals a day suit Pitta.
- Carry dried fruit and nuts for emergencies; this allays the temptation to snack on junk food.
- Eat your main meal at midday and dine as early in the evening as possible, leaving at least two hours between dinner and bedtime.
- Cut down on stimulants, such as hot spices, tea, coffee, and chocolate. Avoid alcohol and drugs, and go easy on red meat and on greasy, pungent, fried, and salty foods.

live seasonally

• Summer produces plenty of cooling fruit: Create some interesting salads.

• In summer, pacify excess Pitta with cooling aloe vera juice.

• The heat of summer is a good excuse to take time out and enjoy the fruit of the last year's labors—relax!

chill out

• Pittas are great planners, but they can overdo it. Avoid the tendency to be overly organized or over-controlling of others.

• Release yourself from rigid timetables.

• Bring spontaneity into your life.

• The world won't fall apart if you occasionally delay work. Put things in perspective—missing a "deadline" doesn't mean that someone dies!

• Let friends and colleagues off the hook occasionally, too.

play fair

• Pittas risk becoming unbalanced by fierce competitiveness. Try choosing sports that are noncompetitive, yet challenging enough that you don't get bored.

• Water sports and winter sports are excellent ways for Pittas to work off excess steam.

• Yoga provides a challenge without being overly competitive *(see pages 160-81)*.

• Partner dancing, such as salsa, makes use of Pitta's coordination and encourages cooperation.

practice nonjudgment

• Schedule frequent periods during which you release yourself from judging anything or anyone. Practice compassion instead.

• Take time each day or week to maintain a receptive silence.

choose cool vacations

• Vacation in places with cool to warm climates. Humid climates are best avoided.

• Don't overplan vacations—take each day as it comes.

• Escape the heat of summer, while satisfying Pitta ambition, by taking a skiing or mountain-climbing vacation.

select the right career

- Executive management, financial advising, law, medicine, and research are good career choices. Pittas are often attracted to, and successful in, high-powered jobs. With such high expectations, you may sometimes experience failure. If so, release yourself from the end result, and consider all you've learned.
- Adopt a cooperative rather than a competitive attitude toward colleagues.
- To balance your strong work ethic and tendency to engage in stressful work, practice relaxation techniques, such as Savasana *(see pages 244–45)* and Meditation *(see pages 250–51)*.
- Take the focus off work by taking an interest in play. Pursue life-enriching subjects, like art, music, dance, and spirituality.

cool your daily routine

- When Pitta peaks at midday, keep calm and cool with Lunar Breathing *(see page 185)*.
- Avoid daytime naps unless in a very hot climate or on vacation, when you might sleep briefly in the shade while the sun at its peak.
- Get plenty of fresh air: Take relaxed walks during the coolest parts of the day.
- Take cool baths, and finish showers with a burst of cold water.

sleep right
• Go to sleep during the Kapha period of the evening—before Pitta takes over at around 10 p.m.
• Use light bed coverings.
• Set up blackout blinds to stop the early summer light from awakening you.

take time out
• Think outside the flurry of short- and medium-term goals every now and then to consider your long-term direction.
• Use regular meditation *(see pages 250–51)* to provide a sense of renewal and enlarge the perspective from which you habitually view life.

ways to throw pittas off balance

- Drinking lots of alcohol
- Eating spicy foods and lots of red meat
- Snacking on salty foods
- Allowing yourself to get worked up, frustrated, and angry
- Exercising at noon
- Using drugs
- Spending time in hot, noisy places
- Striving to win every time, no matter what
- Bottling up your emotions
- Taking regular steam baths and saunas.

the pitta diet plan

To keep the Pitta dosha balanced and achieve ultimate well-being, adopt the following dos and don'ts of good eating. Above all, don't abuse the naturally strong digestion of the youthful Pitta. Preserve it by eating appropriately—plenty of salads; minimal coffee, alcohol, and caffeinated or carbonated drinks. And eat your main meal around lunchtime, when Pitta fire is strongest.

pitta-balancing foods
Pittas tend to have overheated bodies, so choose cooling foods and liquids. Avoid meat, eggs, alcohol, and salt.

pitta-balancing tastes
Sweet, bitter, and astringent tastes are best *(for rasa definitions, see pages 52-55)*; eat fewer pungent, salty, and sour foods.

dealing with vices
If you're a Pitta and want to eat hot, spicy foods, the best times to do so are the morning or evening and the autumn or winter. Avoid these foods in summer or spring, and certainly at midday.

the pitta good food guide

grains
- Barley is an excellent grain for Pittas. Basmati and wild rice, couscous, cooked oats, pasta, and wheat are also suitable.
- Avoid buckwheat, corn, millet, and rye, which have a heating effect on the body.
- Unyeasted breads are better than yeasted.

fruit
- Eat apricots, avocados, cherries, coconut, dried fruit, melons, oranges, and pears.
- Avoid sour fruit, such as cherries, green grapes, kiwi, oranges, peaches, pineapples, and plums. Bananas and papayas should not be eaten regularly.

vegetables
- Pitta types do well with most vegetables. The best choices include broccoli, Brussels sprouts, cabbage, cauliflower, celery, cucumber, peas, squash, and zucchini.
- Avoid tomatoes (sour) and radishes (pungent).

meat and animal products
- Pittas are best advised to avoid meat.
- If you do want to eat meat, chicken and turkey are better than other types.
- Avoid eating seafood, except for freshwater fish, and egg yolks (egg whites are fine).

legumes
- Pittas can digest all types of legumes in small quantities. Garbanzo beans, lentils, mung dal, and tofu are the best choices.

nuts and seeds
- Coconut (and coconut milk) is cooling and beneficial for Pittas.
- Sunflower seeds, pumpkin seeds, and peeled almonds can be eaten occasionally, but other nuts and seeds should be avoided.

dairy
- Limit intake of hard cheeses.
- Avoid sour dairy products, such as yogurt and buttermilk.

oils
- The best Pitta oils are coconut, flaxseed, olive, soy, sunflower, and walnut. Other oils are best avoided.

spices and condiments
• Pittas love spices, but you do best using just the cooling ones: Basil, cardamom, cilantro, fennel, neem leaves, and turmeric.
• Avoid horseradish, mayonnaise, mustard, soy sauce, seaweed, and vinegar.

sweeteners
• Pitta types handle sweet foods better than other doshas do, but avoid white sugar, molasses, and too much honey.
• Substitute fruit juice concentrates, rice syrup, and maple syrup.

alcohol
• Alcohol is heating, so limit your intake to two units a week. Beer is better tolerated than other forms of alcohol.

drinks
• Drink apple, grape, mango, peach, and mixed vegetable juices.
• Rice and soy milks, black tea, and herb teas, including bancha, chamomile, dandelion, fennel, licorice, and peppermint tea, are suitable.
• Avoid coffee and other caffeinated drinks; miso soup; and carrot, grapefruit, orange, sour berry, and sour cherry juices.

pitta menu ideas

These are not complete recipes, but are rather quick ideas for ways to combine ingredients to make the most of the Pitta dosha. Good times of the day and year to eat these foods are also suggested.

seasonal eating
During late spring eat plenty of mangoes, pears, barley, garbanzo beans, mung dal, lentils, cucumber, eggplant, ginger, pumpkin, and zucchini.

During summer eat plenty of apricots, peaches, berries, grapefruit, all melons, mangoes, coconut, squash, turnips, watercress, celery, lettuce, and spinach.

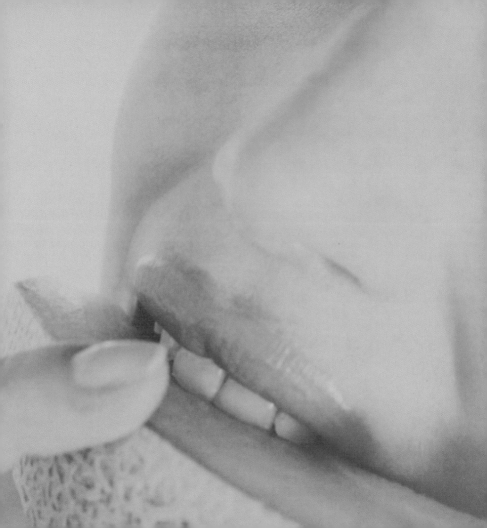

ideas for breakfast

- Oatmeal in winter
- Puffed rice
- Shredded wheat

Accompany the above with cow's milk, soya, or rice milk.

- Whole-wheat muffins
- Whole-wheat toast
- Whole-wheat tortillas.

ideas for lunch

- All varieties of salad (slices of seasonal fruit and pumpkin or sunflower seeds put a nice slant on a plain garden salad)
- Cold bean salad
- Chilled soups in summer
- Tofu burger on a wholemeal bun.

ideas for dessert
- Fruit salad with fresh grated coconut
- Rice pudding
- Tapioca pudding.

ideas for snacks
- Fresh, sweet fruit in season, such as coconut, berries, and red grapes (summer); and pears (fall and spring), or sunflower and pumpkin seed mix (winter)
- Dried fruit, such as apricots, dates, and figs
- Fresh vegetable and fruit juices, with the exception of carrot or sour-fruit juices
- Aloe vera juice in summer.

summer detoxification

Fasting is a key therapy in ayurveda for balancing the doshas. To expel excess Pitta in summer, it's beneficial to take a few days off from work while undergoing a juice fast (see opposite). If you can't stop working but can reduce the amount you work, enjoy a fruit-only fast for a few days, using Pitta-reducing fruit from the list on page 144. If you must keep working, "fast" by cutting out sweet things and sticking to a salad-based diet for 3 to 7 days. Choose vegetables from the list on page 145. Alternatively, you might like to try detoxification with the traditional Indian mildly spiced rice and dal dish, khichadi *(see pages 218–19)*. Any of these fasting options can be combined with use of the triphala blend of herbs (see opposite).

Cautions: If you are under stress, or need to keep working, it is best to wait until a better time arises before fasting. Do not fast, even for a short time, during pregnancy, during lactation, or if you are taking medication. If you suffer from chronic heart disease, diabetes, or another medical condition, obtain clearance first. Consult an experienced natural health therapist or medical practitioner about fasting before commencing a fast. Never undertake a fast for more than seven consecutive days without first seeking professional advice.

triphala

Triphala ("three fruit") is a tonic, made of a combination of three herbs, which regulates all three doshas. The herbs are amalaki (*Emelica officinalis*) to regulate Pitta energy, haritaki (*Terminalia chebula*) to regulate Vata energy, and bibhitaki (*Terminalia belerica*) to regulate Kapha energy. Triphala boosts the metabolism and has a laxative quality that helps clear the body of ama.

Triphala comes in powder form and is taken like a tea after being soaked, or brewed in water. It is also sold as tablets and capsules and can be bought at ayurvedic supply shops. Use every evening after your main meal as part of your detoxification, following the package instructions. While it can be taken for several weeks or months at a time, take regular breaks as its effectiveness lessens as the body adjusts to it. The same cautions apply as with fasting (see below).

following a juice fast

The juice from fruit, without its accompanying fiber, is very high in sugar, so when preparing juices for your fast, mix fruit with vegetable juices. Opt for organic produce where possible. Combinations of the following juices will keep you well hydrated: Aloe vera, apple, carrot, celery, pear, and a little parsley or wheat grass, which helps decrease excess Pitta. Take these juices only for 3 to 5 days, and make sure to get plenty of rest.

massage for pittas

A massage is a great recentering experience for any Pitta type—mobilize toxins from the body by performing a weekly self-massage with oil (follow the simple instructions on page 222). Use Pitta-balancing cold-pressed olive, coconut, or sunflower oil. Pitta people also benefit from Energy-Balancing Massage *(see pages 94–95)* and Easy Abdominal Massage *(see page 223)*, which aids the Pitta digestive fire.

indian head massage

With all those plans for the future whirling around in their heads, Pittas sometimes forget to come back to the body. Indian head massage is the perfect solution—in fact, it brings all dosha types back to base. Massage always feels better when performed by someone else: Swap an Indian head massage with a friend, or give yourself one by following these instructions.

❶ Massage the top of one shoulder (work with the opposite hand for self-massage). Starting at the side of the neck, just near the ear lobe, work down to the tips of the shoulders, squeezing your fingers. Work down the sides of the upper arms to the elbows. Use a slow kneading action. Repeat on the front of the arms.

❷ The person receiving the massage should lean forward, resting the elbows on a table or the lap, forehead in the palms of the hands (rest your forehead in just one hand for self-massage). Massage the back of the neck. Don't apply direct pressure on the spine, but work into the muscles on either side of the vertebrae. Move down from the base of the skull.

❸ With both hands, rub the fingertips around the base of skull. Move upward into the hair until you arrive at the top of the forehead. You can experiment here—try fast frictions over the hair or, with fingers slightly apart, make circles so slow that you feel the skin of the scalp moving over the bones beneath.

❹ With loose wrists and a light touch, let your fingertips ruffle the hair. Then stroke down to the shoulders and tips of the hair. It feels great if you use your fingernails. Starting at the hairline, make frictions downward over the whole face until you reach the sides of the throat. Then cover the face again, making stronger circles. Pay particular attention to the jaw muscles, the temples, and the sinuses at either side of the top of the nose. Finish by pitter-pattering your fingertips like raindrops over the face and closed eyelids.

aromatherapy for pittas

Essential oils can be used to balance each dosha; select those with an aroma that appeals to you. Then create your own aromatherapy treatment by adding a few drops to your bath, oil burner, or pillow pad, or blending them into a massage oil.

Cautions: Do not take essential oils internally, and do not apply them undiluted to the skin. Do not use essential oils while pregnant or breastfeeding: For massage during these times, use the carrier oil alone.

making massage oils
When using essential oils in a blend for massage, use a Pitta-pacifying cold-pressed carrier oil, such as coconut, olive, or sunflower. Add 10 drops total of essential oils (either one oil or a blend of two or more) to 20 ml carrier oil.

aromatherapy oils to uplift pitta
• clary sage • gardenia • jasmine • lavender
• lemon • lemongrass • lime • lotus • peppermint
• sandalwood • vetiver

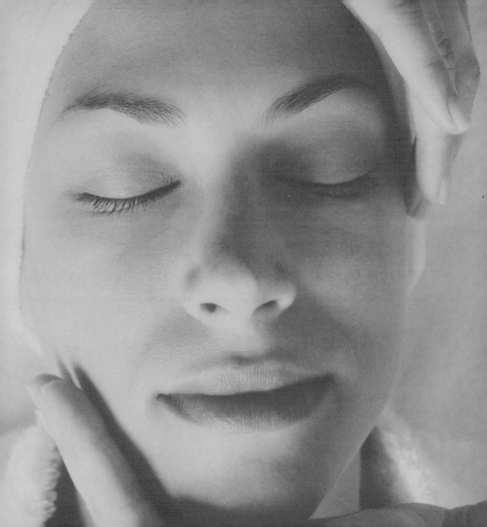

color therapy for pittas

Bringing appropriate colors into your life will harmonize
body, mind, and spirit on a subtle energetic level. For
practical ways to incorporate color into your home,
workplace, and clothing, see page 99, and to introduce
color into your meditative techniques, try the Color
Breathing exercise on pages 190–91.

good pitta colors

- Turquoise, with its cool, refreshing, calming, and soothing qualities, is a useful color for Pitta types. Turquoise balances inflammation and fevers, signs of Pitta aggravation. It also fosters self-containment and can be used by anyone who needs protection from other people's thoughts.
- Magenta is cooling and balancing for Pittas. Since it promotes contentment, it can help balance Pitta ambition, should it become ruthless.
- Yellow brings objectivity when you find yourself overattached to any one idea or desire, and it helps you let go of it, if necessary.
- Indigo and blue are cool colors for fiery Pitta. Blue in particular is a wonderful anti-stress color. Like a long exhalation, it calms, relaxes, and helps an overly busy Pitta sleep more easily.
- Green, neither warm nor cool, brings balance to every dosha and also counters stimulating red, which increases Pitta.

yoga for pittas

As a Pitta with a well-balanced, muscular physique, you can enjoy a rather strong yoga practice, as long as you perform plenty of cooling postures afterward. Forward bends of all kinds, Sarvangasana (pages 114–15) and Halasana (pages 116–17), and Savasana (pages 244–45) all help disperse inner heat.

Many of the postures featured in this section help relieve digestive symptoms and stimulate the digestive fire. They are most suited to balancing Pitta, but you can benefit from any of the yoga poses demonstrated in this book. Simply ensure that the poses are performed in a calm manner, and include plenty of the Pitta-specific poses on the next 20 pages.

Remind yourself not to get competitive—even with yourself. Maintain a diffused general awareness, not forcibly sharp and concentrated, and keep in mind the spiritual side of your yoga practice. You should practice yoga on an empty stomach and avoid eating for half an hour afterward.

breathing for pittas

Yoga breathing techniques help feed the body's vital force for good health and mental stability. In addition, Pitta types benefit from Suryabhedana and Sitali (pages 185–86), which cool the system.

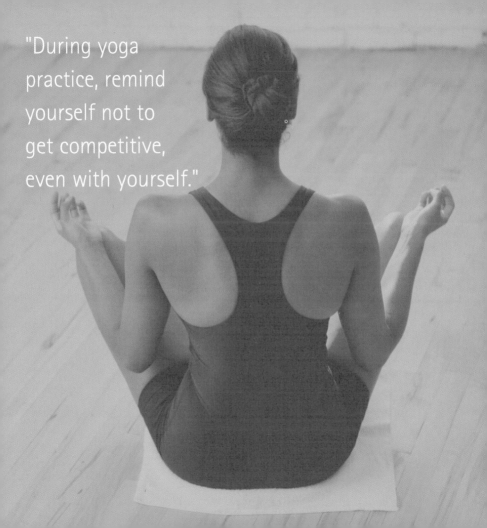

"During yoga practice, remind yourself not to get competitive, even with yourself."

chandra namaskar (MOON SALUTATION)

This sequence is a nice way to start your practice at any time of the day. It enlivens the body during the Kapha morning time. Whenever you choose to practice, let your mind focus on the smooth, enjoyable flow as you connect a single breath with each movement.

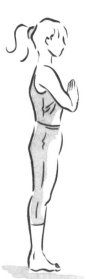

❶ Stand tall, with feet together and palms placed together in front of the chest in Namaste prayer position.

❷ Inhale, and raise the arms overhead. Lift the chest, make a small backbend, and look up.

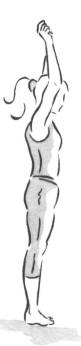

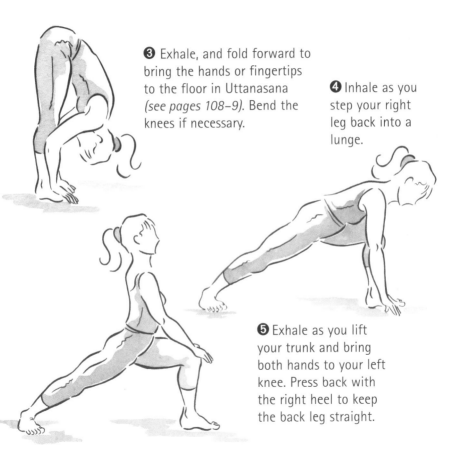

3 Exhale, and fold forward to bring the hands or fingertips to the floor in Uttanasana *(see pages 108–9)*. Bend the knees if necessary.

4 Inhale as you step your right leg back into a lunge.

5 Exhale as you lift your trunk and bring both hands to your left knee. Press back with the right heel to keep the back leg straight.

[163]

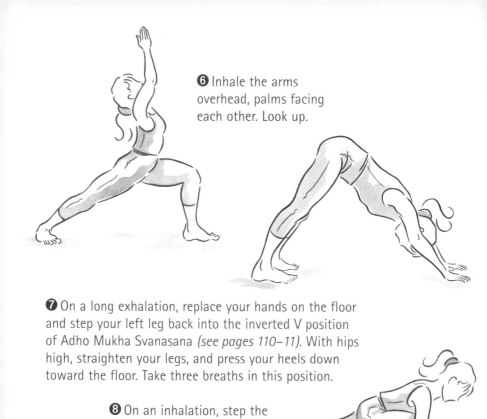

6 Inhale the arms overhead, palms facing each other. Look up.

7 On a long exhalation, replace your hands on the floor and step your left leg back into the inverted V position of Adho Mukha Svanasana *(see pages 110–11)*. With hips high, straighten your legs, and press your heels down toward the floor. Take three breaths in this position.

8 On an inhalation, step the right foot forward between your hands into a lunge, as in step 4.

9 Exhale, step the left leg to the front, and take a forward bend with legs as straight as possible, as in step 3.

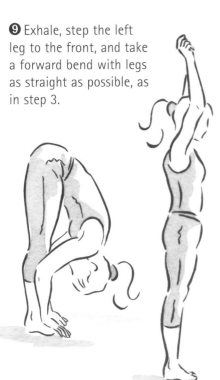

10 With firm abdominal muscles, inhale the arms up and overhead as you come up to standing.

11 Exhale the arms down.

Complete the cycle by repeating all the movements on the other side, taking the left leg back in step 4. Complete three more complete cycles as a warm-up to your yoga practice.

trikonasana (TRIANGLE POSE)

Standing poses simultaneously develop Pitta's even musculature and well-developed coordination. Trikonasana gives a side stretch to complement the other forward and backward bending poses.

❶ Stand with feet wide apart. Rotating from the thighs, turn your left foot and leg in 15 degrees, and turn your right leg and foot out 90 degrees. Check that your feet are in line with each other.

❷ Place your hands on your hips, and square them to the front. Inhale and lift and stretch your arms out to the sides.

❸ On an exhalation, crease in at the right hip, and extend the torso right and down. Place your right hand on your thigh. Make sure that your shoulders don't come forward.

❹ Tuck your chin in a little, turn your head, and look up to your left thumb. Keep your breathing slow and steady as you spread your awareness over your whole body. Come up on an inhalation, and repeat on the other side.

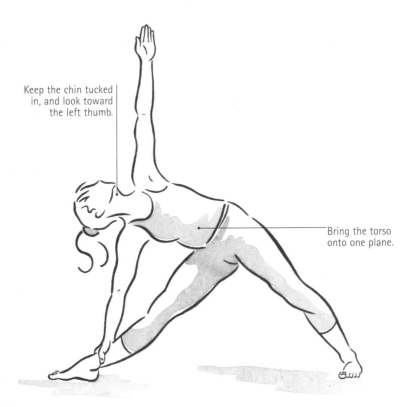

Keep the chin tucked in, and look toward the left thumb.

Bring the torso onto one plane.

parivrtta trikonasana

(TWISTING TRIANGLE)

This revolved version of Trikonasana *(see previous pages)* shares its benefit to the digestive function. Pitta types should follow the Triangle poses with Vrkasana (pages 232–33) and Uttanasana (pages 108–9).

❶ Stand with your feet 3-4 ft. (90-120 cm) apart. Turn your left leg and foot in 60 degrees, and turn your right foot out 90 degrees.

❷ Revolve your torso to the right, then bring your left hip forward to level it with the right hip. Stretch the left arm up in the air, and take a moment to get a sense of the full extension from left ankle to left hand.

❸ On an exhalation, reach the left arm and torso forward and down. Bring the left hand to the floor on the little-toe side of the right foot. Extend the right arm straight up. If you can balance and it feels comfortable for your neck, gaze up to the top thumb. Come up on an inhalation, and repeat on the other side.

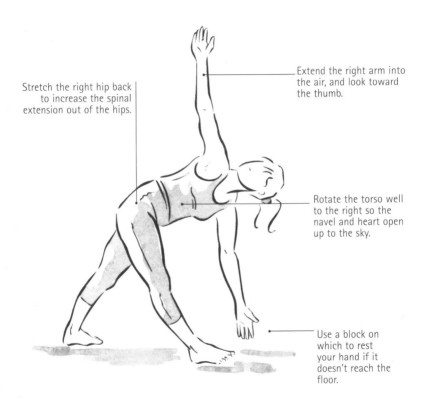

Stretch the right hip back to increase the spinal extension out of the hips.

Extend the right arm into the air, and look toward the thumb.

Rotate the torso well to the right so the navel and heart open up to the sky.

Use a block on which to rest your hand if it doesn't reach the floor.

salabhasana (LOCUST POSE)

This pose nourishes the adrenal glands. If you suffer from back pain, lift just the legs the first time. On the second repetition, keep the feet on the floor and lift only the head and torso. After Salabhasana, further release tension in the abdomen by practicing Dhanurasana (pages 172–73) and Setu Bandha Sarvangasana (pages 112–13).

❶ Lie face down with feet together and arms by your side. Bring your forehead to the floor, and stretch your tailbone toward your feet to lengthen the small of the back.

❷ Tuck your toes under, then lift your knees off the floor, so the legs are straight and the thighs lifting away from the floor. Stretch the heels away for a few breaths, then, on an inhalation, flick the toes away from you and lift both legs up in the air.

❸ Lift the head and chest up from the floor. Bring the arms up parallel to the floor, and stretch them away toward the toes. Hold for five to ten steady breaths. Come down for a short rest, then repeat twice more.

Raise the head and chest, maintaining length in the back of the neck.

Keep the arms parallel with the floor and stretching back toward the toes.

In the full pose, straightened legs are lifted off the floor so you are balancing on your abdomen.

dhanurasana (BOW POSE)

Backbends, by opening up the front of the body, balance the digestive fire. This challenging backbend demands some flexibility in the thighs and shoulders but gives a nice massage to the abdominal organs. After backbends, practice Sarvangasana (pages 114–15) and Halasana (pages 116–17), Bharadvajasana (pages 118–19), and Navasana (pages 122–23), the last of which is helpful for many Pitta-related abdominal conditions.

❶ Lie face down and bend the knees up. Grasp the outer ankles, and bring your forehead to the floor.

❷ Inhale, and lift the knees and thighs off the floor. On your next inhalation, raise your head and chest.

❸ Move the feet up and away to curve the upper body up higher. Let the chest open even more by rolling the shoulders back. Take five to ten breaths before lowering down. Rest and repeat twice more.

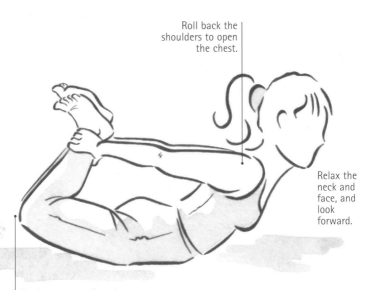

Roll back the shoulders to open the chest.

Relax the neck and face, and look forward.

The knees naturally splay apart, but try to bring them closer to hipbone-width apart: This comes with flexibility.

pashchimottanasana

(SEATED FORWARD BEND)

Forward bends draw the attention inward and are wonderful for Pittas as they cool the body after backbending. Janu Shirshasana (pages 238–39) forms a nice warm up to this pose—Pittas can practice it in a more dynamic way without using a bolster.

❶ Sit with both legs together in front of you. Flex your feet and roll your thighs in toward each other so that the knees and toes face straight up. Inhale, and elongate the torso.

❷ Exhale, and fold forward by hinging from the hips so your navel comes close to your thighs before your chest nears your knees. Depending on your flexibility, hold your shins or the sides of your feet. Stay with the pose for 10-20 breaths, using your arms to lever your torso toward your thighs.

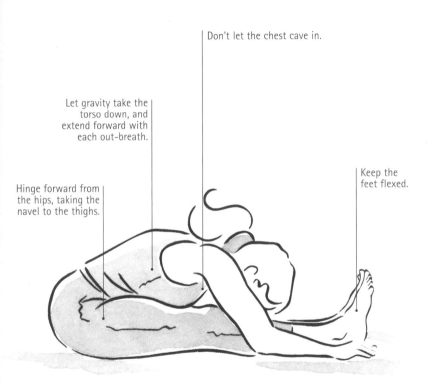

Don't let the chest cave in.

Let gravity take the torso down, and extend forward with each out-breath.

Hinge forward from the hips, taking the navel to the thighs.

Keep the feet flexed.

upavistha konasana

(OPEN ANGLE POSE)

Aside from stretching the inner thighs, this pose brings vitality to the pelvic organs. Reduce the intensity of the stretch should you experience pain in the inner knee.

❶ Sit with your legs about 90 degrees apart. Have your kneecaps and toes facing straight up to the sky.

❷ Press your hands into the floor behind you and, while lifting the chest, tilt the pelvis forward. This movement alone gives a strong stretch on the inner thigh and may be as far as you take the pose for now.

❸ Reach the hands toward the feet and grasp the calves or ankles, or loop the big toes with thumb and index finger. Continue to lengthen from the pubic bone to the top of the breastbone as you exhale forward. Taking care not to round the back, hold for 5-15 breaths.

❹ Inhale to come up, and support your legs under the knees with your hands as you bring them back together.

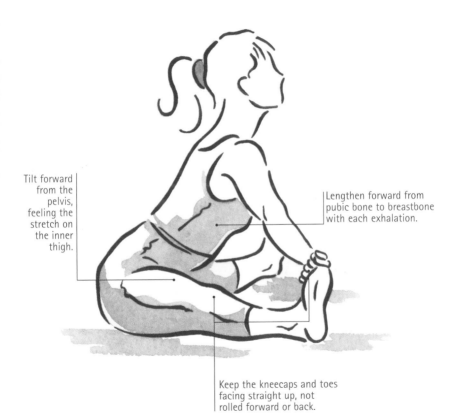

Tilt forward from the pelvis, feeling the stretch on the inner thigh.

Lengthen forward from pubic bone to breastbone with each exhalation.

Keep the kneecaps and toes facing straight up, not rolled forward or back.

supta baddha konasana

(RECLINING BOUND ANGLE POSE)

This restful pose lifts the diaphragm away from the stomach and liver, increases blood supply to the digestive organs, and eases reflux. Use a bolster, or fold up several blankets so they are longer than your torso. The secret of this pose is in finding the right balance between opening the hips and remaining comfortable: If the stretch becomes too intense, it becomes hard to rest.

❶ Sit with one end of the bolster or folded blankets directly behind you, with the soles of your feet together. Bring the heels close to the groin, and let your knees fall out to the sides. To reduce the strain on the inner thighs, place pillows or folded blankets beneath them, if necessary.

❷ Lie back over the bolster. To bring the head higher than the heart, place a small cushion or folded blanket beneath your head. Finally, release your arms out to the sides, palms facing up. Cover your eyes and rest in the pose for 5-10 minutes.

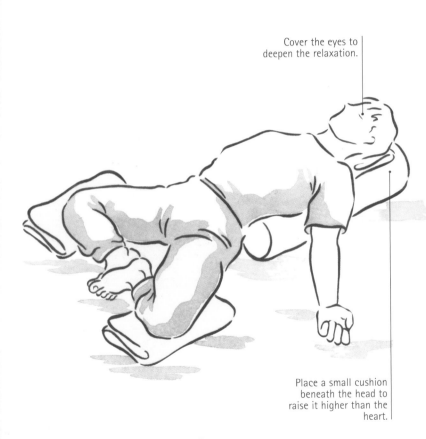

Cover the eyes to deepen the relaxation.

Place a small cushion beneath the head to raise it higher than the heart.

savasana II (BREATHING EASY POSITION)

Like Supta Baddha Konasana (pages 178–79), this elevated yet relaxed supported pose lifts the diaphragm, relaxes the abdomen, and helps diffuse excess heat, making it an excellent asana for Pittas. By opening the chest, it encourages awareness of the smooth, steady breath.

Start by folding one to three blankets to about 8 in. (20 cm) wide. The more blankets, the higher your breathing bed and the stronger the chest-opening action. Experiment with what feels best for you—it should be gentle enough that you can lie quietly and comfortably in the pose for up to 10 minutes.

❶ Sit directly in front of the folded blankets, then lie your torso back over them. Use a cushion or another blanket as a pillow, and let your arms rest out to the sides. Straighten your legs out, and take them a little apart.

❷ Once in position, consciously relax your whole body, from the tips of the toes to the top of the head. Then mentally follow your breath, allowing the exhalations to elongate naturally. Remain in the pose for 5–10 minutes.

completing your yoga practice

All yoga practice should finish with Savasana (pages 118-19). You may keep the blankets as a support as you lie in Savasana, or you may prefer to lie flat on the floor. Practice Savasana for at least 5 minutes for every 30 minutes you have spent performing yoga postures.

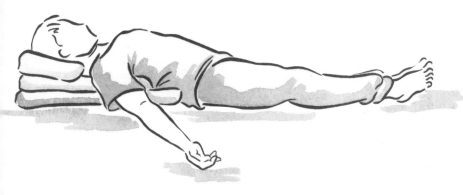

breathing for pittas

Conscious breathing will re-center a Pitta who gets overly caught up in the whirlwind of life. Working with the breath gives the wonderful sense of well-being; a reminder that, even though Pittas tend to continually strive for more, what they have right here and now is to be deeply appreciated.

Once you have mastered this basic technique, move on to one of the two variations of it in Suryabhedana that work more specifically to pacify Pitta and Kapha.

nadi sodhana

(ALTERNATE NOSTRIL BREATHING)

This practice calms those from all doshas, yet leaves them mentally alert. As this breathing balances the nervous system, it settles competitive Pittas who, caught up in their myriad ambitious plans, tend to dwell in thoughts of the future and sometimes need to come back to the here and now. It balances out typical Pitta emotions like irritation, anger, or jealousy. It counters Vata-related feelings of being uptight, anxious, or confused. Practice at sunset and sunrise is a good time for Vata. Practice before bedtime helps those suffering insomnia float off to sleep.

quieting the mind

❶ Sit up straight on your heels, cross-legged, or on a chair. On your right hand, tuck the index and middle fingers into the palm, in Krishna Mudra. Inhale fully through both nostrils.

❷ Close the right nostril with the thumb of the right hand, and exhale fully through the left nostril. Then inhale through just the left nostril.

❸ Close the left nostril with the ring and little fingers of your right hand, release your thumb, and exhale through the right nostril. Inhale through the right nostril. Then close the right nostril with the thumb, release the left nostril, and exhale through the left nostril. This is one cycle.

❹ Complete three to seven continuous cycles, before lowering your arm and taking some slow, quiet breaths through both nostrils. This is one round. When you feel ready, start the next round. Let the air flow through the nostrils at a constant rate. There should be no strain; let a soft quality come to your breath. Complete three rounds in all, then finish by relaxing in Savasana (pages 118-19).

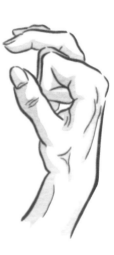

To use the whole hand, put the knuckles of the index and middle fingers above the bridge of the nose between the eyes. Ring and little fingers block the left nostril, thumb the right.

variations: suryabhedana

pitta-pacifying lunar breathing

While the right nostril relates to the warming sun energy, the left is linked to the cooling lunar energy. As this cooling breathing activates the parasympathetic nervous system, those of any dosha may benefit in times of stress. Using the right hand to open and close both nostrils in turn, breathe in only through the left nostril and out through the right each time. Build your practice to three rounds of three cycles in all.

vata- and kapha-pacifying solar breathing

This version of Nadi Sodhana warms the system, and helps balance the coolness of vata and kapha. Activate the heating solar energy by breathing in only through the right nostril and out only through the left. Build your practice to three rounds of three cycles in all.

sitali (COOLING BREATH)

A thirst-quenching breathing technique, this is helpful in the heat of summer or whenever Pitta needs pacifying. As it is cooling, Sitali is less often practiced during the Vata autumn or Kapha winter. The technique works by sucking air in across moisture on the tongue to cool the body and reduce thirst, and was used by yogis in the desert in ancient times. The method involves sticking the tongue out, making a round hole with the lips, and curling up the edges of the tongue into a funnel.

❶ Sit comfortably erect. Exhale through the nose, then, on opening your mouth, poke out your tongue, and turn the sides up and in toward each other to make a strawlike channel. If you find this impossible, like 25 percent of people, just keep the tongue flat.

❷ Take a long, slow inhalation, drawing the air in through the curled tongue. Hold the breath, take the tongue in, close the mouth, and exhale through both nostrils. Repeat for ten more rounds and, over a couple of weeks, build up to 20 cycles.

visualization for pittas

Determined and clear thinking Pitta types well understand the power of the mind. Enjoy a short mental holiday with these visualizations. Emerging refreshed, people can then tackle their daily tasks with renewed vigor.

sanctuary visualization

A sanctuary is a place where you feel completely safe, protected, and nurtured. Use the technique that follows to help you find that place within, adopting or adapting the idea given below for your dosha, to help balance your bodymind.

❶ Sit comfortably or lie down. Visualize yourself in an unspoiled natural setting, perhaps the one suggested for your dosha. Let yourself hear the sounds of the animals, and take in the natural smells of your special place, as you connect to the essence of nature in this welcoming retreat. Infuse yourself with the harmonizing feel of this peaceful and enriching haven. Relax.

❷ To end the visualization, open your eyes, and sit quietly. Know that your sanctuary is always there when you need it. You just need to take time to access it.

- **pitta ideas**

You might be sitting beside a mountain stream, in the dappled sunlight under the cool forest canopy. As you absorb the calming sound of the trickling water nearby, smell the fresh, pure, clean air. Among the sounds of the forest animals in the background is the call of distant birds. Listen to the soothing sounds of the gentle wind in the trees, and feel a great calmness well up inside you.

- **vata ideas**

You might be sitting in the sun by a beautiful, still pond. Feel the sunlight on your skin and on your closed eyelids. Inhale the warm air, heavy with the scent of the lush trees nearby. In this safe and nurturing place, any animals are friendly, curious, and unafraid. You feel perfectly peaceful.

- **kapha ideas**

You might be walking slowly along the shore of a beach. Under the warm sun, listen to the sound of the waves rolling in. Smell the invigorating, fresh salt air. As you take in the gentle call of the seagulls in the background, feel the breeze in your hair and against your skin.

color breathing

Use color to re-harmonize the system and bring healing vibrations to energize areas of weakness. Choose a color to which you feel intuitively drawn. It might be one of the colors recommended for your dosha in the chart opposite, or you might choose white light, which brings clarity. Note the qualities and effects of the color on your mind and body and remember its complementary shade.

❶ Sit comfortably or lie down. Inhale through the nose, and visualize yourself breathing in your chosen color. As you exhale through the nose, visualize yourself breathing out its complementary color.

❷ From your nostrils, let your color inhalation travel down to your chest into the vertebral column. With each breath, the color intensifies. It strengthens all the more as you exhale its complementary shade.

❸ When the spine is densely filled with your color, let it filter out through your body. Make sure any areas that need healing are filled with this color energy, especially the heart center. Before you complete the exercise, mentally seal your color—and its particular qualities and effects—into your body. To end the visualization, open your eyes, and sit quietly.

inhale	visualize the color	qualities	doshas	effects	exhale
red	like a rose	vitality, energy, willpower, courage, warmth, assertiveness	vata, kapha	warming	turquoise
orange	like an orange	joy, fun, creativity, optimism, tolerance	kapha	warming	blue
yellow	like a flame	uplifting, intellectual strength, objectivity, wisdom	pitta	warming	blue
green	like grass or a forest	cleansing, balancing, recharging by harmonizing	vata, pitta, kapha	neutral	magenta
violet	like the twilight sky	insight, intuition, self-respect, dignity	vata, pitta	cooling	yellow
magenta	like flower petals	release from obsessional thoughts or preoccupation with the past	vata, pitta, kapha	cooling	green
turquoise	like crystal-clear water	anti-inflammatory, fever-reducing, boosting to the immune system	vata, pitta, kapha	cooling	red
blue	like the deep ocean	relaxation, peace, sincerity, organizational abilities, anti-insomnia	pitta, kapha	cooling	orange

vata rhythms of fall and early winter

After summer, changeable temperatures and dry falling leaves herald the arrival of the Vata season. With its cold, erratic winds, fall is a busy period of reorganization—a time of high energy and increased activity. It is a productive period when the Vata energy helps us achieve our goals, just like the other animals, who scurry to complete their tasks before winter.

vata

"Vata is sometimes called the king of the doshas: It moves before the others."

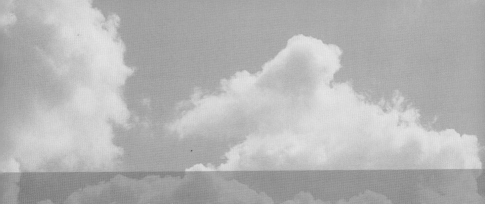

contents:

the characteristics of vata

Vata energy is a combination of the elements air and space. Often compared to the wind, the Vata nature is erratic and changeable. The wind is quick, cooling, and drying, and Vata people often lack moisture and dislike the cold. Space, like the sky, has transparent, dispersing qualities, and this relates to the lightness and mutability of the Vata character. When in balance, Vata individuals are joyful, sensitive, and exhilarated; they are artistic, enthusiastic, and imaginative, full to the brim with so many ideas that they have trouble remembering them all.

the vata body

Either very tall or very short, Vata people are physically light and wiry. The typical Vata face is long and angular, with a long, thin neck. Compared to others of their own ethnic background, Vatas have darker skin, and their hair is often dark, coarse, curly, or wavy. Eyes may be close-set, small, or asymmetrical. Teeth tend to be irregular and can be small, or else large and protruding or angular. Characteristics caused by variability in the bones, such as pigeon toes, bow legs, a sway back, a deviated nasal septum, or weak teeth, are more signs of the presence of Vata.

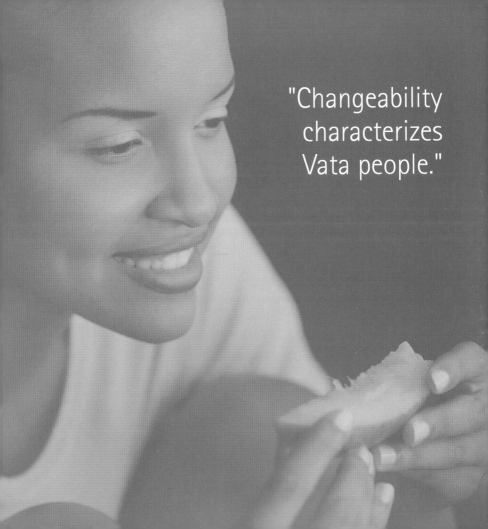

"Changeability
characterizes
Vata people."

the vata season

Autumn, with its crisp, cold weather, is Vata season, a time of high energy, unpredictable weather, and increased activity—and chapped lips and dry eyes. One Vata time of day is from midafternoon to dusk, a productive period when the Vata energy helps us to complete our tasks before the day's end. Vata also arises in the cold predawn hours and is strong until daybreak, when Kapha takes over.

the vata pace of life

Vatas have a great enthusiasm for life and happily involve themselves in new projects. In their bursts of exuberant energy, they are quick to pick up on fresh ideas. If their imaginative selves are not actually setting the trends, they will at least be the first to adopt the latest ones. Vata powers of concentration could be stronger, and while Vata people grasp new concepts quickly, they don't always remember them some time down the road. Vatas are generous and believe money is for spending. Being spontaneous, they spend freely on trifles, and find it hard to save.

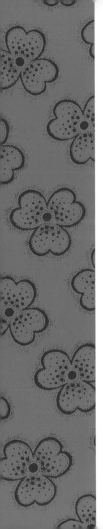

Vata types like to do everything quickly, preferring to be physically active and on the go, partly because that's their nature, partly to ward off boredom. Vatas are fast to react, even if they are not always correct in their responses. They often make decisions in haste and repent at leisure and have outbursts that are easily forgotten (by them, if not by others). Excitable by nature, Vatas tend to fidget, and they often bite their nails when nervous. They don't have strong roots and tend to be very mobile, changing houses, jobs, or cities more often than others. Vatas think of sex often, and, with a powerful imagination, have an active fantasy life. Although Vatas are easily aroused, they have less stamina than Pitta or Kapha types, both of whom have stronger sexual needs.

vatas and change

Although they do best with regularity in eating, sleeping, working, and resting, Vatas prefer change to routine. They thrive on plenty of stimulation in every aspect of life, from fitness routines to work to social life. Vata people delight in having friends from all walks of life, and they are great company, being funny, quick-witted, and charming. With their transitory nature, Vatas love travel, but unfortunately it depletes them.

vata energy levels

Vatas have a lack of stability that can manifest in changeability in everything: Friendships, opinions, emotions, memory. They love new hobbies and take to them quickly, often leaving their last project unfinished. Being impulsive by nature, Vata types tend to overexert themselves, and keep little energy in reserve. Periodically, energy reserves run out, and Vatas get so exhausted that they need to rest.

vatas and warmth

Possessing a naturally cold, dry body type, Vatas have cold hands and feet and constantly need to be warmed—they are always the first to request extra blankets on the bed. They love the sun and feel more alive after basking in its rays. A Vata needs warmth not only in climate, but in food and drink. Vata types have a healthy appetite, although they tend to bolt their food, and the force of their digestive system changes from day to day.

the vata sleep habit

Vatas sleep the least of the three doshas, and as they age (and Vata increases with age in everyone), they sleep even less. Their sleep is easily disturbed, particularly as Vatas dislike noise at any time. Vata people are at their peak in the morning.

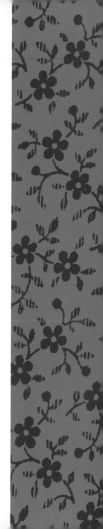

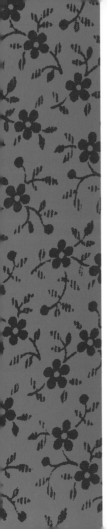

vatas and weight

Changeability characterizes Vatas, and their weight can fluctuate throughout life. Those who seem too thin and have trouble gaining weight manifest a great deal of Vata. Generally though, Vatas have a slight build and of all the doshas, they find it easiest to stay slim and lose weight.

the vata time of life

Each dosha has an affinity with a particular time of life. Vata reigns over the years after 60, when most people notice that their systems feel drier and they need less sleep. During old age, although the body is moving toward death, wisdom never stops growing, and the spirit can soar, too. The Vata stage of life is a time to benefit from your accumulated wisdom and enjoy the fruits of what you have learned during your life.

symptoms of aggravated vata

- worry, fear, and anxiety
- disturbed sleep
- reduced ability to focus
- envy
- dissatisfaction

how to balance vata

The Vata type needs to compensate for a weak digestive fire, feed the body with warmth and moisture, and adopt routines in every part of life. The following tips may help you toward these goals, but when it comes to implementing change, do it gradually. Don't completely overhaul your lifestyle from one day to the next, particularly your diet—food affects the mind more than you might think.

eat fewer foods more often

• Four small meals a day are generally better than three large ones for Vata.

• The more types of food the digestive system encounters at once, the harder it has to work. Since the Vata digestion tends to be weak, Vatas thrive by eating fewer varieties of food at a single sitting.

• When several foods are cooked together, as in a soup or a stew, they are easier to digest. Vatas do very well on one-pot meals enhanced with a few warming herbs and spices.

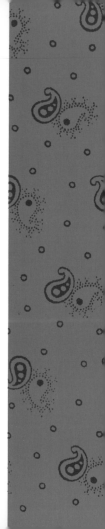

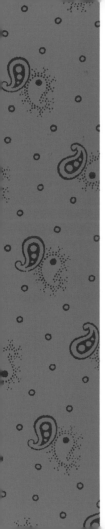

keep hydrated

- To keep the body hydrated and detoxified, drink plenty of herbal teas and warm or tepid water between meals.

- Drinking water during meals dampens the digestive fire, especially if the water is cold or iced. If you must drink at mealtime, sip small quantities of warm water.

- While hydrating the body, eat plenty of fiber to counter the Vata tendency toward constipation.

eat seasonally

- Eat according to the seasons—price is a good guide to which foods are in season.

- During autumn, pacify Vata by eating plenty of cooked root vegetables and having regular massages.

nurture your body

- Eat warm, moist foods.
- Oil your skin several times a week *(see pages 220–23)*.
- Book a regular massage as part of an overall commitment to slowing down and treating yourself lovingly.

take warm baths

- Enjoy warm to hot baths. Light candles and take time just for you so that you emerge feeling calm and soothed.
- Steam baths are also good for Vatas, especially in the autumn and the late afternoon.

establish routines

- Wake up, go to sleep, and eat meals at the same time every day. If you stay regular in all habits, you are less likely to exhaust yourself and will be better able to enjoy your naturally fast-paced life.
- Insert rest breaks throughout your daily routine for yoga stretches and deep, slow breathing.

choose the right career

- Creative work feeds the Vata soul. Vatas do well in jobs that require creative thinking, such as advertising, public relations, marketing, writing, fashion, art, music, and film, especially if they don't have too many deadlines!
- In your downtime, pursue calming hobbies such as gardening. Arts and crafts are another wonderful channel for creative Vata energy.
- If you feel you can't change a very erratic part of your life: Working in a super-fast-moving job, freelancing, or shift working, or having to

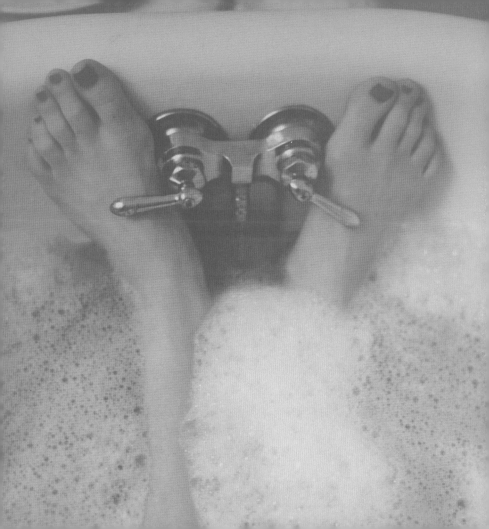

travel—be sure to counter it with a Vata-pacifying diet *(see pages 210–13)*. Try to fill your leisure time with slower, emotionally restful activities.

exercise gently

• Although Vatas love vigorous exercise, regular gentle exercise is actually better for them. Exercise based on controlled movement and discipline is ideal—try T'ai chi or yoga, in which your mind is fully absorbed in your actions.

• Around dawn, when Vata is dominant, you need calming, warmth, and moisture, even more than usual. This is a good time to practice Vata-balancing yoga postures, breathing exercises, and meditation *(see pages 250–51)*.

• Sit in silent meditation each day. If possible, choose the same time of day and the same location. Schedule time in your busy Vata calendar and stick to it.

focus

• Don't let your mobile Vata mind stop you from concentrating.

• Focus on one thing at a time instead of juggling tasks and people and skipping from one thing to another.

honor your space
• Create a safe, calm, secure environment at home and work. Turn the space you inhabit into a sanctuary that truly nourishes you.
• Surround yourself with soothing, soft music.

try napping
• Ayurveda tells us it's best not to sleep when the sun is out, but of all the doshas, Vatas can best afford to sleep during the day. Ideally, practice Savasana *(see pages 118-19)* for 20 minutes each day.
• If you really need sleep, take just a 20-minute nap. Lying on the floor in Savasana will prevent you from sleeping too long.

choose chill-out vacations
• Take your vacation in a single place rather than moving around a lot.
• A nice vacation mantra for Vata is sun, sea, and sleep!
• Choose a warm location, enjoy going slow, and resist the urge to cram every minute with activities.
• Be aware that traveling, particularly flying, aggravates Vata.
• During trips and after you arrive, keep warm and well hydrated.

give thanks

- When you find yourself becoming anxious, remind yourself to be grateful for what you have: Your health, sustaining food, a loyal pet, a friend to confide in.
- Consider your cup half full rather than half empty.

stay quiet

- Loquacious Vata benefits from practicing silence. Take some time each day for solitude. Not talking, even for just 15 minutes, brings you back to yourself.
- Make time every day to commune with nature. Appreciate the natural world during a slow walk, or sit and contemplate a beautiful view. This special time is a way to check in with yourself and keep yourself aligned with the changing seasons and the overall direction of your life.
- Vatas are very sensitive to noise, so sleep in a quiet place.

ways to throw vatas off balance
- Eating lots of cold foods, frozen foods, and leftovers
- Bolting food on the run
- Keeping an irregular lifestyle with no routine
- Fasting
- Worrying
- Missing sleep
- Keeping feelings bottled up
- Freelancing or working night shifts
- Working in a job with constant interruptions
- Traveling a great deal
- Playing fast-paced computer games and going to loud, flashy nightclubs
- Stimulating the body with drugs, refined sugar, and lots of alcohol
- Taking part in adrenaline-rush sports, such as bungee jumping.

the vata diet plan

In general, in order to achieve ultimate well-being, Vatas should minimize their intake of raw foods; eat plenty of warm, moist foods; and cut out caffeine and anything sugary. Vatas do well on four small, regular meals a day rather than three large ones—and they should eat their evening meal well before bedtime.

vata-balancing foods

As Vata has light, dry, and cold qualities, the natural foods to balance excess Vata are those with heavy, oily, warming qualities. To avoid aggravating Vata, steer clear of dry foods, such as toast, dry cereals, or dried fruit; cold food such as ice cream; and iced drinks.

vata-balancing tastes

Choose sweet, sour, and salty foods *(for rasa definitions, see pages 52-55)* and eat fewer pungent, bitter, and astringent foods.

dealing with vices

If you choose to eat refined and processed foods, don't do so in Vata-increased times of the day or year—early morning, late afternoon, or fall. The safest time to indulge is the late morning, and the safer seasons are spring and summer.

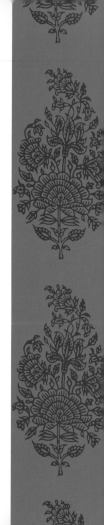

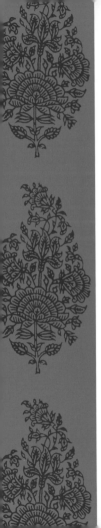

the vata good food guide

grains
- Eat oats and all types of rice and wheat.
- Eat less barley, corn, couscous, millet, muesli, puffed cereals, and yeasted breads.

fruit
- The best varieties of fruit for Vata are heavy, wet, and sweet, such as mangoes, peaches, or bananas.
- Fruit eaten raw is cooling; fruit that is stewed or otherwise cooked helps warm Vata.
- Avoid dried fruit and limit intake of apples, melons, pears, and astringent fruits, such as cranberries and pomegranates.

vegetables
- Cooked vegetables are preferable to raw for Vatas.
- Avoid frozen or dried vegetables. Don't eat salads straight from the fridge; warm the ingredients to room temperature first.
- Vegetables to eat more often include artichokes, carrots, green beans, leeks, pumpkin, squash, sweet potato, and zucchini.
- Vegetables to eat less often include broccoli, cabbage, cauliflower, eggplant, mushrooms, and raw onions.

meat and animal products

- Vatas are well suited to a diet that includes meat, and on a psychic level meat can help ground them.
- Beef, duck, and fish are better than chicken, lamb, and pork.
- Vatas who don't eat meat do well with eggs.

legumes

- Vatas have difficulty digesting legumes; make sure they are soaked beforehand and well cooked.
- The easiest legumes for Vatas to digest are mung dal. Lentils, garbanzo beans, and tofu can be eaten in small amounts.
- Adding sea vegetables, such as kombu, to a legume dish lessens flatulence—to which Vatas are prone.

nuts and seeds

- All nuts and seeds are fine, especially those made into moist nut butters or nut milks.

dairy

- Vatas generally manage dairy products well.
- Hard cheeses are less desirable than soft cheeses, and cow's milk is better than goat's milk.

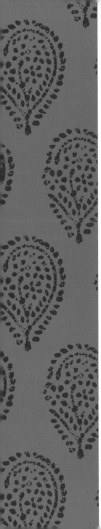

oils
• All oils are fine, but the best choice is sesame oil.

spices and condiments
• All spices except caraway are good, but don't overdo them; be especially careful with hot spices, such as chili peppers and horseradish. Vatas should eat cayenne and fenugreek only in moderation.

sweeteners
• Avoid white sugar.
• Substitute fruit juice concentrates, honey, molasses, or occasionally maple syrup.

drinks
• Drink wine in moderation, but not if it has chemical additives. Avoid beer and spirits.
• Vatas tend toward dryness and need to keep their systems well hydrated. Rice and almond milks, miso soup, carrot juice, and most fruit juices are good. Herb teas (cinnamon, chamomile, fennel, fresh ginger, licorice, and peppermint teas) are useful, too. Avoid astringent herbal teas, such as those made with nettle or sage. Skip caffeinated drinks, carbonated drinks, and apple and cranberry juices.

vata menu ideas

The ideas below are not complete recipes but are rather quick ideas for ways to combine ingredients to make the most of the Vata dosha. Good times of the day and year to eat the suggested foods are also listed.

seasonal eating
During fall, eat plenty of rice, wheat, mung dal, peas, cucumber, pumpkin, squash, and zucchini.

ideas for breakfast
- Porridge
- Puffed brown rice
- Shredded wheat

Accompany all above with freshly stewed fruit and cow's milk, rice milk, or almond milk
- Hot herbal teas, especially fresh ginger tea, or warm milk
- French toast
- Buckwheat pancakes
- Scrambled eggs with sautéed onion and a little chili powder.

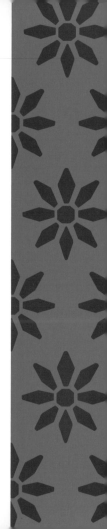

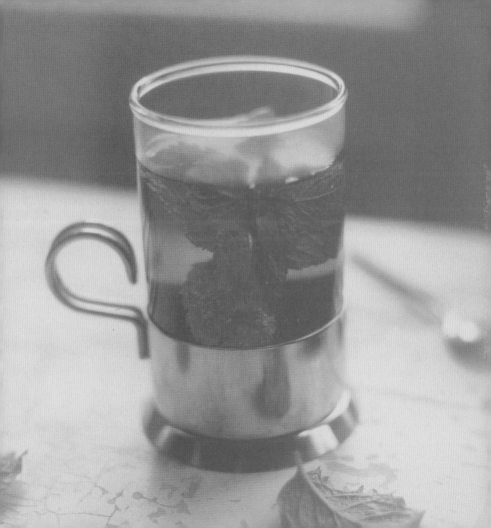

ideas for lunch
- Khichadi (see overleaf)
- Rice with a sauce of spicy mixed seasonal vegetables
- Mung dal and vegetable one-pot meals
- Hot soups with mung dal or seasonal vegetables
- Wholemeal sandwich with avocado and cheese, egg salad, or tahini spread.

ideas for dinner
- Khichadi (see overleaf)
- Casseroles and stews
- Soups and chowders
- Rice noodle dishes with vegetables and a little tofu
- Creamy, or occasionally tomato-based, pasta dishes
- Side salad.

ideas for dessert
- Rice pudding made with spices (cardamom, cinnamon, cloves, ginger)
- Crepes with stewed fruit
- Pumpkin pie
- Warm fruit cobbler.

autumn detoxification

The Vata autumn in India, when the weather is neither too hot nor too cold, is a traditional time for fasting. In chilly climates, this purification is a preparation for eating more to ward off the external cold of winter. Spring, when all living things emerge from winter hibernation, is another good time to undergo seasonal detoxification, as the digestive fire is weaker then. Khichadi, a stew of basmati rice and split mung dal, is a vital element in ayurvedic nutritional healing. Both basmati rice and mung dal are tridoshic foods—balancing to all three doshas—and in combination they are a source of complete protein. One-pot meals are also extremely beneficial for anyone at a time of weakness—during an illness, when recovering from illness, or during detoxification.

Although spring is an obvious time for an internal spring cleaning, khichadi is balancing and sustaining enough to be eaten at any time of the year. This warm, mildly spiced, soupy dish is excellent for aggravated Vata during the Vata-dominated autumn season. See overleaf for instructions on using khichadi as part of a do-it-yourself detoxification. You may also like to combine a khichadi diet with the triphala blend of herbs *(see page 153)*.

basic khichadi

In this simple khichadi recipe on the facing page (preparation time: 1 hour), vary the vegetables and spices according to your dosha and taste as follows:

Vatas: Add a mix of any of the spices in the ingredient list and try also combinations of asafetida, black pepper, cardamom, cinnamon, cloves, and fennel. The only spices to limit are caraway, cayenne, and fenugreek.

Pittas: To the ingredients listed, feel free to add combinations of cinnamon, mint, and saffron. Avoid anise, asafetida, basil, cayenne, cloves, mustard seeds, nutmeg, oregano, and paprika.

Kaphas: Omit the fennel and salt; instead try combinations including asafetida, basil, black pepper, caraway, cardamom, cayenne, cinnamon, dill, and fenugreek.

ingredients and method for making khichadi

1 tablespoon ghee (clarified butter) or olive oil
2 bay leaves
1 teaspoon of each: Cumin seeds, fennel seeds, ground
   cilantro, sea salt, fresh grated ginger root, turmeric
1 cup organic basmati rice
1 cup organic split mung dal, presoaked for 3 hours
4-6 cups of purified water
2 oz. (60 g) diced organic carrots or celery
Fresh lemon juice
Chopped cilantro leaves

❶ Melt the ghee or oil in a large pan. Add the cumin, bay leaves, fennel seeds, ground cilantro, salt, and ginger, and sauté for 1-2 minutes.

❷ Add the turmeric, rice, mung dal, and 4 cups of water. Bring to a boil. Boil for five minutes uncovered, stirring occasionally. Cover, and cook for 25-30 minutes, adding more water if necessary to maintain a soupy consistency. Add the carrots or celery, and cook for another 15 minutes. To serve, add lemon juice and garnish with cilantro leaves.

massage for vatas

Oil massage holds a special place in Indian life. Traditionally, infants and young children are massaged every week, and adults regularly massage their bodies. Massage stimulates blood and lymph circulation and detoxifies. Ayurvedic oils—made by decocting ayurvedic herbs for many hours in base oils—are considered powerful medicine. When applied to the skin, they not only moisturize but are absorbed into the body and balance the doshas. You can obtain specific dosha-balancing oils from ayurvedic doctors or ayurvedic supply shops.

Massage is a marvelous treatment when aggravated Vata leaves you feeling dry, uptight, and frazzled; Vatas are grounded and soothed by regular massage. Book a regular oil massage with a massage therapist—for Vata, this is a necessity rather than a luxury—and, in between, oil yourself as often as possible: Three times a week is good. Vatas also enjoy Indian Head Massage *(see pages 154–55)* and Energy-Balancing Massage *(see pages 94–95)*.

choosing oils to suit your dosha

Any oil can be used to counter the drying effects of Vata. Sesame, avocado, castor, and flaxseed oils are Vata-specific. Apricot kernel oil, jojoba, and the rather expensive wheatgerm oil are suitable for all doshas. Since oil is absorbed by the skin, use cold-pressed organic oils.

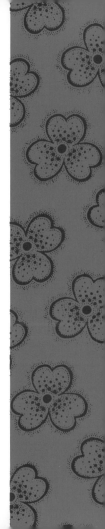

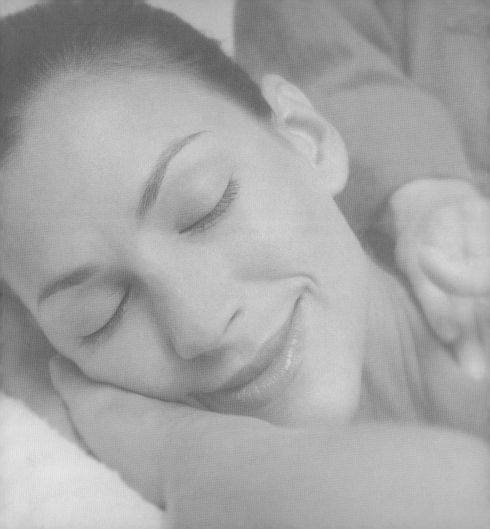

self massage with oil

The best time to give yourself an oil massage is before your morning shower. Work with an oil appropriate for your dosha *(see page 224 for Vata, page 156 for Pitta, and page 96 for Kapha)*.

❶ Sit naked on a towel and begin applying oil by massaging the soles of the feet, then every part of the feet.

❷ Work up one leg, massaging in the direction of the heart. Then massage the other leg in the same way.

❸ Now oil your hands, and massage up each arm toward the shoulder.

❹ Oil the back and front of your torso. Here, you can massage in any direction you prefer.

❺ Oil your throat, neck, and face. Finally, rub a little oil into the scalp and the tips of the hair.

❻ Wait for ten to twenty minutes to let the oil soak in before showering. Ideally, this should be a quiet time to relax and reflect.

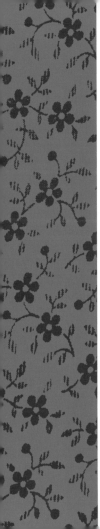

easy abdominal massage

A quick-fix massage for a Vata comprises work on the abdomen. This massage eases colic and wind and counters the constipation to which Vata is prone. As this massage tones the abdominal organs, all doshas benefit from treating themselves to a tummy rub. Remove belts and loosen tight waistbands. If you want to use an oil, use one appropriate for your dosha *(see page 224 for Vata, page 156 for Pitta, and page 96 for Kapha)*.

❶ Lie on your back. Bend your knees and lean them in on each other so that the abdomen is relaxed. Place both hands flat on your abdomen and start by making large, slow circles over the whole area.

❷ Move to the lower right side of the abdomen. Use the fingers of both hands to make small, slow circles as you move up the right side to press in just under the ribs.

❸ Move across the abdomen, massaging below the ribs and just under the ribcage.

❹ Finally, work down the left side of the abdomen. Massage around this clockwise circuit a few more times, then lie still and relax.

aromatherapy for vatas

Essential oils may be used to balance each dosha—select those with an aroma that appeals to you. Add a few drops to a soothing warm bath or steam treatment, place them on an oil burner or pillow pad, or blend them into a massage oil.

Cautions: Do not take essential oils internally or apply them undiluted to the skin. Do not use essential oils while you are pregnant or breastfeeding. For massage during these times, use the carrier oil alone.

making massage oils
When using essential oils in a blend for massage, use a Vata-pacifying cold-pressed carrier oil, such as sesame, avocado, castor, or flaxseed. Add 10 drops total of essential oils (either one oil or a blend of two or more) to 20 ml carrier oil.

aromatherapy oils to uplift vata
• camphor • cedarwood • cinnamon • eucalyptus
• frankincense • geranium • juniper • lavender • lemon
•myrrh • neroli • patchouli • rose • rosewood • sage

color therapy for vatas

Color is a wonderfully health-giving and noninvasive treatment. As each color in the spectrum has its own vibration, thoughtfully chosen colors help balance the system in every way.

Try the following exercise: To energize water with a beneficial color, wrap colored cellophane around a glass jug filled with water. Place it in the sun for a few hours, then sip solarized water that has imbibed the vibrations of your color.

good vata colors
- Red is warming, stimulating, and energizing. It gives willpower and extra follow-through Vatas need to bring ideas to fruition.
- Blue is a relaxing color. It brings peace and helps reduce insomnia.
- Magenta is an integrating color with a harmonizing force.
- Green is balancing for all three doshas and helps counter the indecision many Vatas experience. As a more static color, green calms Vata's tendency toward excess movement.
- Yellow relates to the element air. Warming yellow is Vata-increasing, so yellow in excess can increase Vata anxiety, leading to nervousness and shallow breathing.
- Violet relates to the Vata element of ether. It's helpful to an unsettled Vata as it calms the body and balances the mind.

yoga for vatas

Vata people tend to be slim, and either very flexible or very inflexible. They tend toward postural imbalances more than the other doshas do. Vata disturbance leads to posture problems, including scoliosis, bow legs, and rounded backs, so Vatas benefit greatly from the following body-balancing postures, especially when they are practiced with a calm, focused mind. Continued yoga practice also helps allay the stiffness Vatas experience with age.

Vatas should adopt a slow, steady approach to yoga asanas. You need to build endurance, so rather than moving in and out of poses, try to hold each one for some time, with mental concentration. Take care not to exhaust yourself; instead, work on building a grounding and nurturing practice slowly and steadily.

The routine suggested for your dosha type might be your basic one, but when seasonal or lifestyle changes affect your bodymind balance, do bring in elements of the yoga routines suggested for the other doshas (for Pitta, see pages 160-79; for Kapha, see pages 100-23). For example, in Kapha-dominated winter, when it's hard for everyone to get off the sofa, Pittas and Vatas also benefit from Sattva Namaskar (pages 230-33).

Having said this, it's a good idea to finish with postures appropriate for your constitution. For Vata, forward bends, a nice long Savasana *(see pages 244–45)*, breath work, and meditation are ideal *(see pages 250–51)*. When busy, Vatas find it hard to make time for practice; remember that it's better to do fewer things slowly and with awareness than to move quickly and automatically through many poses.

"Adopt a slow, steady approach to your yoga practice."

sattva namaskar

(SALUTE TO INNER CALM)

This sequence focuses and steadies the mind. It can be practiced on its own whenever you feel you need to come back to yourself. Practiced at the beginning of your yoga session, it can clarify your intent and set the tone for your practice. Take three or four long, slow breaths in each position before moving to the next one.

❶ Sit on your heels and put your palms together in Namaste prayer position, so that your thumbs are at your breastbone.

❷ On an inhalation, raise your arms up and touch both wrists to the crown of the head. Ease the elbows back and let the heart center (the center of the chest) open.

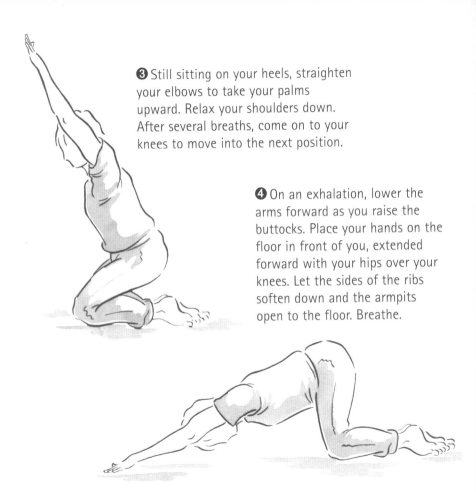

❸ Still sitting on your heels, straighten your elbows to take your palms upward. Relax your shoulders down. After several breaths, come on to your knees to move into the next position.

❹ On an exhalation, lower the arms forward as you raise the buttocks. Place your hands on the floor in front of you, extended forward with your hips over your knees. Let the sides of the ribs soften down and the armpits open to the floor. Breathe.

sattva namaskar

(SALUTE TO INNER CALM)

❺ Slide your hands in toward you and form a diamond shape with thumbs and forefingers. Ease your buttocks down to your heels and rest your forehead in the diamond. This pose, or a similar one with arms draped around the body so the fingers lie near the toes, is a relaxing pose for Vata at any time.

❻ With middle fingers pointing forward, straighten your elbows so that the weight is resting on your hands and gaze at the floor in front of you. Let the front of the torso, as well as the back, lengthen. Hold, breathing. Come back to sitting on your heels.

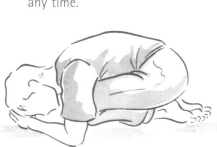

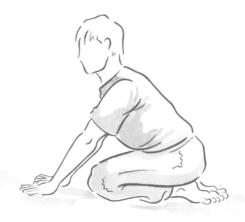

7 Bring your hands back to Namaste prayer position and have the sides of the thumbs meet the third-eye area, the space between the eyebrows.

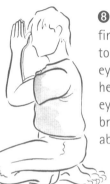

8 Bring your fingertips down to touch between the eyebrows, bow your head, and close your eyes. Remember to breathe from your abdomen.

9 Lower the hands in Namaste to their starting position by the heart, and repeat two more cycles as you salute your inner tranquility.

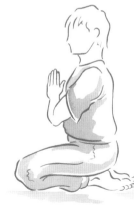

vrkasana (TREE POSE)

Balance poses are as much about settling the mind as physical coordination. Flighty Vatas will benefit from concentration on maintaining a steady balance. Vatas also benefit from other standing poses, such as Parivrtta Trikonasana (pages 168–69), an unwinding balance, and Uttanasana (pages 108–9).

❶ Stand with your feet together and let your weight settle through the soles. Bend the right leg slightly and feel your full weight through the left foot. This grounding pose allows you to establish a good connection to the earth, so take a few breaths as you open yourself to it.

❷ Grasp your right ankle, and place the sole of the right foot against the left inner thigh. Press your foot against your thigh, and your thigh against your foot.

❸ When you feel stable, let both arms float up overhead, and press the palms together. The key to balancing is to maintain perfect concentration and a calm mind. Hold for eight steady breaths before calmly coming down, recentering, and practicing on the other side.

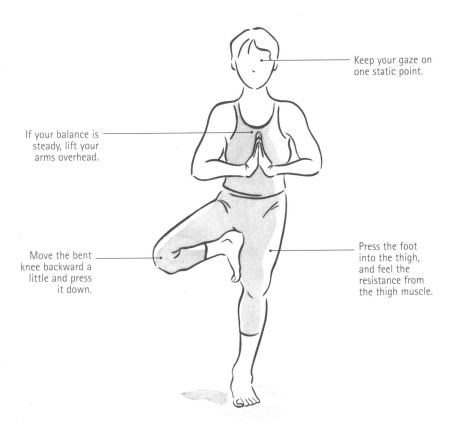

Keep your gaze on one static point.

If your balance is steady, lift your arms overhead.

Move the bent knee backward a little and press it down.

Press the foot into the thigh, and feel the resistance from the thigh muscle.

bhujangasana (COBRA POSE)

This pose counteracts the Vata tendency toward rounded shoulders. Its abdominal stretching effects work against menstrual irregularities and constipation. After this pose, practice Salabhasana (pages 170-71). Vatas tend toward poor circulation, so try inversions such as Sarvangasana (pages 114–15) and Halasana (pages 116–17), which also counter constipation. Follow these poses with Bharadvajasana (pages 118–19), to unwind a tense Vata.

❶ Lie on your front with your feet together, and place your hands on the floor under your shoulders so the fingertips are level with the tip of the shoulders. Your elbows will be in the air.

❷ Press the shoulders away from the ears so that they move toward your hips; bring your elbows closer together. Press the pubic bone down to lengthen the back of the waist.

❸ Keep the length in the lower back; lift your head and shoulders. Gaze forward and upward. Hold for five to eight breaths before coming down to rest. Repeat twice more.

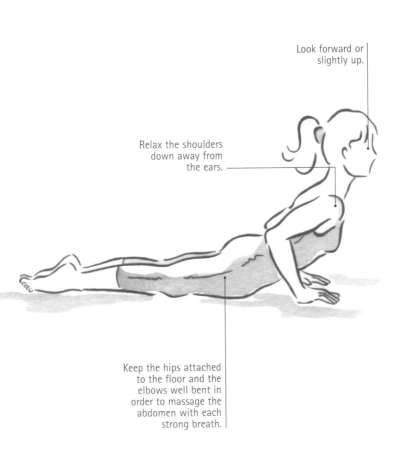

Look forward or slightly up.

Relax the shoulders down away from the ears.

Keep the hips attached to the floor and the elbows well bent in order to massage the abdomen with each strong breath.

eka pada pavanamuktasana

(WIND-RELIEVING POSE)

Placing a gentle pressure on the abdomen, this sequence of stretches relieves cramping, bloating, constipation, and gas, to which the Vata person is prone.

❶ Lie on your back. Inhale, curl your upper body up, draw your left leg in, and hug it close to your chest. Draw the nose to your knee.

❷ Exhale, lower the leg, return the head to the floor, and rest. Repeat with the right leg, then perform eight more rounds.

❸ Finally, hug both legs into the belly. With head and shoulders resting on the floor, rock slowly from side to side, letting the warmth and pressure of the thighs sink into and massage the abdomen.

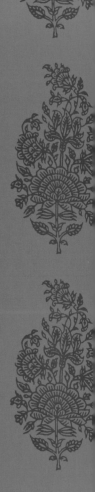

Draw the nose to the knee.

Move slowly and rhythmically in time with your breath.

Press the lower back to the floor.

[237]

janu shirshasana (SEATED HEAD-TO-KNEE)

Forward bends help ground an airy Vata, encourage pelvic circulation, and draw the senses inward, even more so when performed with a bolster-like support. To make a bolster: Roll several blankets up, or use some sofa cushions. Practice Pashchimottanasana (pages 174-75) and Upavistha Konasana (pages 176-77) in the same way. To ease menstrual cramps, bloating, or abdominal discomfort, try this variation: Roll up a blanket tightly, to a diameter of about 3 in. (7.5 cm). Push it into the crease of the hips as you fold forward.

❶ Sit with your legs in front of you. Bend the right knee out to the side, and bring the sole of the foot in line with, but not under, the left inner thigh. Place the bolster on your outstretched leg.

❷ Inhale, and stretch your arms up to lift out of the hips. Exhale and fold forward, bringing your arms on top of the bolster. Rest your forehead on the bolster, using extra blankets to increase the height of the support if your forehead doesn't reach down. Rest for 1-2 minutes. As you release forward, slide the bolster toward your foot.

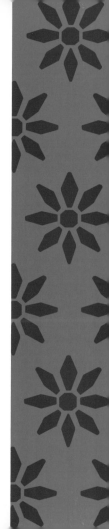

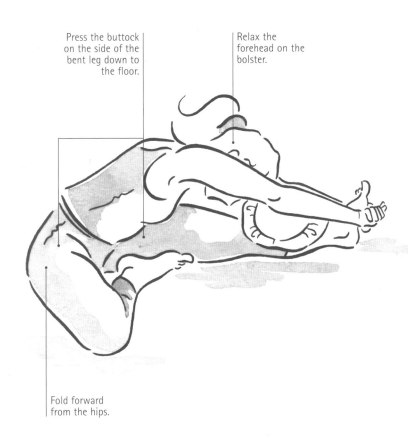

Press the buttock on the side of the bent leg down to the floor.

Relax the forehead on the bolster.

Fold forward from the hips.

supta balasana

(BELLY-SOOTHING RESTING POSE)

Here, a lovely gentle pressure on the abdomen relieves cramping, bloating, constipation and gas. Use the mind-body connection as staying physically still, and notice how it helps an overactive mind to quiet.

❶ Fold a blanket into a 5 in. (12.5 cm) wide pad that is longer than your torso. Roll up one end of the pad, and lie with your abdomen over the roll. The blanket should end just below your throat, and your forehead should come naturally to the floor, where it rests comfortably.

❷ Experiment with the position of the blanket roll. It should feel nurturing. If you desire, place a heat pack or hot-water bottle under the abdomen, so the warm, damp heat can soothe the Vata energy. Stay, gently rocking or moving, as long as it feels good.

Move your pelvis slowly
to find your perfectly
comfortable position.

Let your mind linger
on the sensations in
the belly.

Observe how the breath
slows and steadies as you
settle into the pose.

yogamudrasana

(SEALING POSE)

Mudras are yoga positions that work with the vital force and seal it internally. This pose quiets the mind noticeably and provides a soothing pressure to the abdomen.

❶ Sit on your heels. Grasp your left wrist with your right hand behind your back.

❷ Inhale, and extend the front of the torso upward; then exhale and fold forward, bringing your forehead to the floor.

❸ If you find that your buttocks sit high in the air rather than near the heels, if you have high blood pressure, or if your forehead doesn't easily reach the floor, raise your head a little higher and support it on a folded blanket. Let your whole body relax, and stay in the pose as long as comfort allows, mentally following the breath.

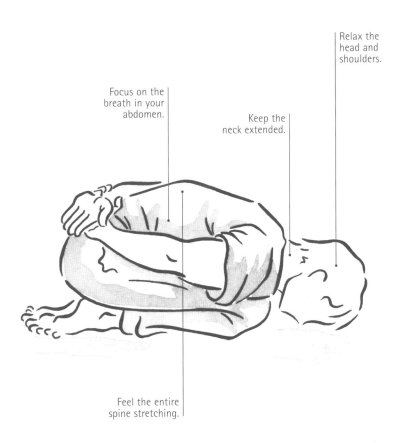

Relax the head and shoulders.

Focus on the breath in your abdomen.

Keep the neck extended.

Feel the entire spine stretching.

savasana (CORPSE POSE)

Always finish your yoga session with Savasana. This relaxation pose allows the body to settle and the effects of your yoga practice to consolidate. It is a very important pose for Vatas, but all doshas need to finish their yoga practice with this asana. Cover yourself to keep warm. If you have back pain, bend the knees up and keep both feet flat on the floor.

❶ Lie on your back with feet apart and flopped out to the side. Keep arms at the sides of the body, palms facing up. Make sure your body, including the position of your head, is symmetrical. Close your eyes.

❷ Feel your bones become heavy, and let the relaxation sink deep into your body. Release any tension. Relax your mouth and tongue. Relax your eyelids and eyeballs deep into your skull. Feel the skin on your face smooth and soften as you relax even further.

❸ Lie relaxed for 10-20 minutes. As your body releases, note how it feels heavier. Observe the breath as it becomes more delicate. Feel the heart center opening.

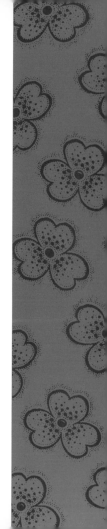

When it's time to come out of Savasana, gradually deepen your inhalation and run your thumbs over your fingertips. When you are ready, roll over onto your side. Take your time coming up to sit. Resist the temptation to be sucked into the frenetic pace of life again, at least for a while. Stay centered and relaxed as you go about your tasks.

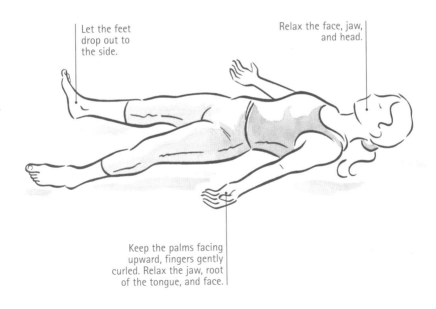

Let the feet drop out to the side.

Relax the face, jaw, and head.

Keep the palms facing upward, fingers gently curled. Relax the jaw, root of the tongue, and face.

breathing for vatas

There are few ways as efficient to quiet the mind as becoming completely absorbed in the breath. The following two techniques bring your awareness to the sound of the smooth and steady breath. As yogis have known for centuries, evenness in the breath leads to evenness of temperament. Vatas also derive great benefit from practicing Nadi Sodhana (pages 182–83), and Uddiyana (page 125).

ujjayi (WARMING BREATH)

As a warming breath, Ujjayi is very useful to reduce Kapha and Vata, especially during fall and winter. During its practice, the glottis in the throat is constricted. As the air flows past it, friction is produced, which is heating to the system. You can use the Ujjayi breath during your posture practice, too.

❶ Sit comfortably upright. Breathe in through the nose and out through the mouth, making a long "haaaa" sound, as if you were trying to fog up a mirror. This partially closes the glottis (the part of the throat that closes when you gargle water).

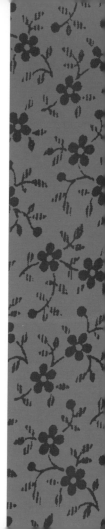

❷ After a few rounds, close your mouth midway through an exhalation, but continue to make the "haaaa" sound with your lips together. It will become a soft sound, like a "hmmm" that you can feel in the back of the throat.

❸ When you feel comfortable with this, continue to make the internal "hmmm" sound even with the inhalation. Once you have mastered continuous breathing through the nose, let this thin breath be soft. Even the breath so that it becomes long, clean, and steady. Practice for 2 minutes, and gradually lengthen the duration.

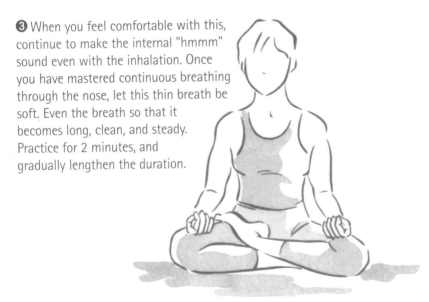

bhramari
(BEE BREATH)

Making a sound on the exhalation brings constancy and length to the breath and gives a point of focus for the mind. As you become absorbed in the internal vibrations, you will experience a deep soothing of the mind. Should you experience dizziness or tingling, or if your mind becomes agitated, switch to regular breathing.

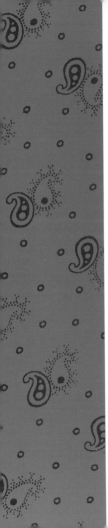

❶ Sit on a rolled-up blanket with knees bent up in front of you. Place your elbows on your knees. From here, bring your palms up to cover your eyes and, with your thumbs, press on the little flap that closes over the ear holes.

❷ Press your tongue lightly to the roof of the mouth. When you exhale, make a humming noise. After a long exhalation, take a slow, patient inhalation and, as you make the next low-pitched, constant hum, feel the vibrations in the soft palate of the mouth.

❸ Continue breathing and humming in this way, feeling the vibrations spill from the mouth up into the skull. Become absorbed in the vibrations as they spread down from the throat into the rest of the body.

❹ Practice Bhramari for 2 minutes, over time building up to 5 minutes. Afterward, sit or lie quietly with eyes closed to enjoy the soothing aftereffects of the vibrations in the body and mind.

meditation

Because meditation brings us back to ourselves, people of every dosha benefit from its practice. The natural time for meditation is after you have loosened your body with some stretches, enabling you to sit perfectly still. Traditionally, sunset and sunrise are considered ideal times for meditation. Trataka *(see overleaf)*, Bhramari (pages 248–49), and Nadi Sodhana (pages 183–84), are helpful exercises to still the mind before meditation.

basic meditation

❶ Choose a comfortable sitting position with back and neck erect. Start by observing the flow of air through your nostrils and the sensations created by each inhalation and exhalation.

❷ Observe any thoughts that arise. They will float into your consciousness: Just let them float away again. Refrain from getting caught up in judging anything. Should you find yourself following a train of thought, gently and kindly bring yourself back to observing the rhythm of your breath in a detached way.

❸ After spending some time with your breath like this, you may like to direct your mind toward a single thought, perhaps contemplation of concepts such as love, freedom, peace, and so on. If you choose a subject, remain an detached observer, watching the thoughts around your topic arise and drop away again.

❹ To end the meditation, open your eyes and sit quietly. Bring the meditation into your daily life by staying attuned to your thoughts, words, and actions, all of which affect those around you.

VATAS ALSO BENEFIT FROM THE FOLLOWING TECHNIQUES:
energizing visualization, SEE PAGES 126–27,
color breathing, SEE PAGES 190–91,
AND sanctuary visualization, SEE PAGES 188–89.

trataka (STEADY GAZING)

This technique develops concentration and leads the mind toward a meditative mindset. It is best practiced after sunset, with the lights turned off. Place a candle on a low table so that when you sit in your comfortable erect position, its flame is at eye level. Close your eyes and steady your breathing. After a while, open your eyes and move your gaze from floor to candlestick to candle flame. Gaze steadily at the flickering flame. Often the eyes may sting or water, but resist the urge to blink.

❶ Begin by holding for at least 30 non-blinking seconds, and build up your gazing time to 1 minute. After the first round, close your eyes and sit quietly, allowing the afterimage of the flame to float in your mind's eye. When it has faded, open your eyes for a second round of gazing.

❷ This time, focus on the blue part of the flame. Again, don't let yourself blink—it becomes easier with practice. Take a second rest period.

❸ Repeat again, this time gazing at the whole flame and observing the dancing particles. While you stay focused on the flame, "widen" your vision out so that it may include even the walls to the side of the room. Afterward, again sit quietly with closed eyes until the afterimage fades.

❹ Finally, rub your palms together vigorously, building heat from the friction. Place your hands over your eyes and let the warmth enter your lids to soothe and recharge your eyes.

the year's close

You may have noticed how one positive lifestyle change naturally seems to lead to others. A dietary improvement may pave the way for a new exercise regimen, which in turn might encourage a more positive mental outlook.

If you follow the guidelines in this book through the four seasons of the year, you will have the chance to ponder *why* you want to be healthy. You don't need to seek perfect health for its own sake, but so that you can actively live a full, productive, helpful, and vibrant life. With the tools of *The Ayurvedic Year*, you can be the best possible you.

Your body is the vehicle you have been given to carry you through life, and it feels better to be in a healthy body than in an unhealthy one. Put simply, it feels good to feel good! By following the guidelines in this book—perhaps adopting a well-regulated diet, or practicing a daily yoga routine that works for you—you will feel cleaner and stronger and will be living better than you did in the past. Sometimes you may feel that certain areas of your life and health need fine tuning. But your inner trust will continue to grow, and your capacity to intuit and respond to your own needs will continue to improve. Ultimately, you will be able to fully embrace and enjoy the journey we call life.

resources

Fawley, David
Yoga and Ayurveda
Lotus Press, 1999

Lonsdorf, Nancy
A Woman's Best Medicine: Health, Happiness, and Long Life Through Maharishi Ayur-Veda
JP Tarcher, 1995

Morrison, Judith H.
The Book of Ayurveda: A Holistic Approach to Health and Longevity
Fireside, 1995

Svoboda, Dr. Robert
Ayurveda for Women: A Guide to Vitality and Health
Inner Traditions, 2000

Tiwari, Bri Maya
The Path of Practice: A Woman's Book of Healing with Food, Breath, and Sound
Ballantine, 2000

Vasant, Lad
The Complete Book of Ayurvedic Home Remedies
Three Rivers Press, 1999

Warrier, Gopi and Gunawant, Deepika
The Complete Illustrated Guide to Ayurveda
Element Books, 1997

The Ayurvedic Institute: www.ayurveda.com
Maharishi Ayurveda Products International, Inc.: www.mapi.com